MILK PRODUCTION AND PROCESSING

Authors

Dr. C. Ibraheem Kutty is post graduate in the subject of Animal Reproduction and is presently holding the post of Assitant Professor at College of Veterinary & Animal Sciences, Thirssur under Kerala Agricultural University. Having completed Veterinary graduation in 1992, he had worked as Veterinary Surgeon under Animal Husbandry Department, Kerala and subsequently joined university service. Besides qualifications in Veterinary science, he is unique in having post graduation in medical science as well, completing Master of Public Heath course from Sree Chitra Thirunal Institute for Medical Sciences & Technology, Thiruvananthapuram-a deemed university and referral hospital of top ranking at national level.

During his professional career, he was holding the charge of Professor and Head of a major research station under Kerala Agricultural University for about 15 months. He could also work as guest lecture for Vocational higher secondary courses, took part in lot of extension and training activities and presented research paper in few international and many national conferences. He has more than 30 research papers in his credit published in international journals, internet and Indian journals. He has published one book and many popular articles in Malayalam as well.

Sheeba Khamber is wife of Dr. C. Ibraheem Kutty and is holder of B. Tech. degree in Dairy Science & Technology from Kerala Agricultural University. Graduated in 1998 she was involved in dairy development activities as Dairy Extension Officer and continues in the post under Government of Kerala. She has also worked as guest lecture for vocational higher secondary course for 2 years and that service was prompted this venture of preparing a comprehensive textbook on the subject.

MILK PRODUCTION AND PROCESSING

by

Dr. C. Ibraheem Kutty
B.VSc. & A.H.; MVSc; MPH

Sheeba Khamer
B. Tech. (Dairy Sci. & Tech.)

2014
Daya Publishing House®
A Division of
Astral International Pvt. Ltd.
New Delhi – 110 002

Published by   : **Daya Publishing House®**
                          A Division of
                          Astral International Pvt. Ltd.
                          – ISO 9001:2008 Certified Company –
                          4760-61/23, Ansari Road, Darya Ganj
                          New Delhi-110 002
                          Ph. 011-43549197, 23278134
                          E-mail: info@astralint.com
                          Website: www.astralint.com

Laser Typesetting   : **Classic Computer Services**
                          Delhi - 110 035

Printed at   : **Thomson Press India Limited**

PRINTED IN INDIA

CONTENTS

Chapter 1
INTRODUCTION TO DAIRY FARMING

Dairy sector in India has the major responsibility of providing milk to growing population, ensuring animal protein in their diets and thus ensuring better health. Among farm animals dairy cows and buffaloes are major producers of valuable human foods such as milk and meat and thus plays vital role in improving the nutritional status of people especially in villages. The raw materials for this are mainly wastes and by products of agriculture and other industry enabling its effective utilisation, reducing disposal burden and at the same time converting into highly nutritious human food.

Present Scenario

Dairy Sector in India is formed of around 60 million cattle and 40 million buffaloes, reared by about 70 million farmers. These animals produces about 80 million tonnes of milk every year making India the No 1 producer of milk in the world. Even then per capita availability of milk at present is only around 215 g/day, while WHO has recommended a per capita daily consumption level of 280 g/day for better health. Also demand for milk further increases with rapid growth of human population and standard of living necessitating urgent measures for increasing milk production in the country.

India leads other countries with respect to number of cattle, buffaloes and goats as shown below. In order to increase milk production, we cannot further increase the number of dairy animals as there is shortage of land and other resources even now. It is important to bear in mind that 80 million metric tonnes of milk is produced in India to become No 1 milk producer is from around 100 million dairy animals. While in USA - the second major producer of milk in the world, nearly 78 million metric tonnes of milk is produced every year from roughly one quarter of total cattle and buffalo population in India. This indirectly points to very low productivity of our animals and inferior management. Hence possible ways to achieve production hike include increasing productivity of animals through scientific breeding and management.

Table 1

Species	Present Population in India (In millions)	Proportion of World Population	Approximate World Population (Millions)
Cattle	210	15 %	1400
Buffaloes	75	50 %	150
Goats	110	20 %	550

Proportions of milk contributed by various dairy animals in India are as follows.

Table 2

Buffalo 52 %,	Cattle 45 %	Goat and others 3 %

Buffaloes contribute major share of milk produced in the country even though population of buffalo is only 2/3 as that of cattle. This is attributable to the possession of best dairy breed of buffaloes in the world such as Murrah and Surti, which forms major proportion of buffaloes in the country. For the same reason there is less scope for rapid improvement of productivity from buffaloes when compared to cattle. Most of the cattle belong to non-descript breeds, which are very poor yielders compared to buffaloes, exotic breeds of cattle and crossbred cattle. Approximate daily productivity (expressed in litres) of each type of dairy animals in India are as follows:

Table 3

Non Descript Breeds	Crossbreds	Indian Milch Breeds	Exotic Dairy Breeds
Cattle			
1-2 litre	6 - 8 litres	4 - 6 litres	20 -30 litres
Buffalo		**Goats**	
Dairy breeds	Others	Indian milch breeds	Others
4 - 5 litres	2 - 4 litres	1-2 litres	0.5 - 1 litre

Since majority of cattle in India belongs to non-descript (local) breeds, which are poor yielders, total milk production from cattle is lower than that from buffaloes. But there is lot of scope for improving productivity of local cattle breeds incorporating germplasm of high producing exotic breeds. Such efforts were going on many years and have contributed considerable hike in production.

Dairy Development Programmes

Programmes were included in the five-year plans of India for the planned development of dairy sector and upliftment of dairy farmers through improvement of animals, increasing availability of resources and providing marketing facilities. Some of the major programmes were

Key Village Scheme (KVS)

Launched during the first five year plan (1951 - 1956) at different parts of India with the objectives of cattle improvement, fodder production and immunisation of animals against major diseases. The programme was made operational through 6 key village blocks, under them there were key village units, each covering 2500 cattle. During second plan period number of Key village blocks were increased to 10 and the activities were expanded.

Operation Flood Programme (OFP)

This was started during fourth plan period (1969 - 1974) and was the major multipurpose scheme launched by the union ministry of agriculture in the dairy sector. The programme was originally proposed by National Dairy Development Board (NDDB) and was approved by FAO (Food and Agriculture organization -United Nations) as part of its World Food Programme (WFP). The programme was also designated as "White Revolution" and was aimed at establishing a broad base for dairy industry in India.

OFP-1

Launched in 1970, with the main objective of capturing market for milk especially in four metro cities. Initially 1160 million rupees were generated through sale of milk powder and butter oil gifted by WFP and was used for establishment of co operative societies so as to improve milk marketing facilities. At the end of first OFP there were 13000 APCOS (Anand Pattern co operative societies) under 39 district level milk unions. This resulted a three fold increase in procurement of milk from villages within 10 years ensuring regular supply of milk and regulating price in metros.

OFP-2 & 3

OFP 2 was started in 1978 and OFP 3 in 1987 and were continuation of OFP-1. The main objectives were increasing milk production through improvement of cattle and buffaloes aimed, (1) to meet the high demand for milk, (2) increasing the nutritional status and income of village community, (3) establishment of infra-structure required to support a viable dairy industry and (4) establishment of national milk grid connecting major cities and production centres. By the end of OFP-3 there were 70000 APCOS in 170 milk sheds with over 93 lakh dairy farmers as members spread over 270 districts of India.

Dairy Farming

Dairy farming is the primary occupation of a good proportion of farmers in India. Dairying also forms major subsidiary occupation of those with other primary occupations especially agriculture. Dairying and crop production are mutually integrated since both are interdependent and benefited each other. The importance of this is further increased upon realisation that more than 50 % of farmers involved in dairying are marginal and land less farmers and agricultural labourers. Thus dairying forms the livelihood of weaker sections through enabling landless farming and providing reasonable income throughout year.

Importance of Dairy Farming

Dairy farming forms very important production activity especially in villages for the following reasons.

1. Production of highly nutritious food materials. Milk and milk products forms the most important and best source of animal protein in the food for human beings. Milk is a nearly complete food supporting better growth rate and is very important in the diet for growing children, sick and elderly.

2. Dairy animals utilizes cheap roughages which are not directly utilized by man, in order to produce high quality food materials such as milk and meat. Besides effective utilization of household and agricultural wastes and by products, dairying also minimizes the problems of waste disposal.

3. Dairying provides employment to a considerable proportion of population especially to ladies. For most farmers involved in crop production, dairying forms the subsidairy occupation. More over surplus family labour can be effectively utilised. When large volume of milk is made available, its processing and manufacturing of various products can generate large number of employment opportunities.

4. High market demand for milk makes disposal easier and makes dairying a source of regular cash income. Unlike crop production seasonal fluctuations are minimal for milk price and it gives subsistence income during the off seasons of crop production.

5. Major groups of farmers involved in dairying are small farmers and agricultural labourers. Hence it is an occupation of poor and land less people providing them a means for "land less agriculture". Dairying also plays a vital role in improving the nutritional status of their families.

Advantages of Dairy Farming

Dairying has got so many advantages over agriculture and other occupations. Some of the major advantages are the following :

1. Highly nutritious food materials are produced from cheap roughage and concentrates, which are other wise unutilised. Grasses, hay and straw forms the major

roughage, and concentrates fed to dairy animals consists of oil cakes and agricultural by products like bran. These items are not used for human consumption hence does not cause any competition with human beings for food items. Dairy animals being ruminants, have highest efficiency of utilising roughage and in return they produce highly nutritious food items such as milk and meat.

2. Dairy farming is mutually integrated with crop agriculture, utilising by products of crops and providing highly valuable manure or bio fertiliser for conserving soil fertility and thus supporting crop production. Manure adds organic compounds to soil, which helps to maintain humus, aeration and growth of beneficial micro-flora in the soil. Through grazing or addition of dung, nutrients lost from the soil are made up and soil fertility is conserved.

3. Milk and meat being highly nutritious food materials containing all the essential nutrients required to support maximum growth rate. Household production of milk improves nutritional status of family members, provides manure for house hold cultivation, utilises house hold wastes and enables effective utilisation of leisure time of family members.

4. Milk and products have good market demand especially in urban areas enabling easy marketing. Surplus milk produced in villages can be easily converted into milk products which have good nutritive value and demand. Hence the producer will not have much problem for marketing products of dairying.

5. Initial investment required for starting a small dairy unit (household dairying) is small and there are lot of agencies providing financial support for dairy enterprise. Hence it is easy to start dairy enterprise as a means of employment

6. Unemployment problem is more in rural areas and dairying being rural based provides better employment opportunities in villages either in the form of milk production or product units. One or two cows can be maintained even with minimum land availability. Hence it can be accepted as a means of occupation for unemployed youth, elderly and even ladies.

7. While income from most of the crops is seasonal, income from dairying can be obtained throughout the year, thus forming a source of subsistence income even during non-harvest seasons. Hence integration of crop and dairying helps to eliminate seasonal scarcity of agricultural families.

8. For agricultural labourers, unemployment during non crop seasons can be ensured through dairy animal production.

9. Dairying forms insurance against crop failure, since even if crop fails due to some unforeseen reasons, diversification of agriculture with dairying helps the farmer to earn some income and thus to make up the loss to some extent.

10. Animals forms a type of readily disposable income source, which can be used in case of some emergencies, moreover under optimum management animals multiplies faster enabling rapid multiplication of capital.

Limitations of Dairy Farming

Even though dairying has got various advantages, there are some limitations as well such as:

1. *Confining job*: Dairying requires long hours of work every day without any interruption. The cows has to be milked twice or thrice daily at fixed timings depending upon the marketing and other conveniences, along with regular feeding, washing, shed cleaning and so on. Hence alternate arrangements has to be made for taking few days off, or going away or even while falling sick. Getting suitable person for replacement is also not that easy.

2. Dairying requires varying degrees of skill for different activities, and some amount of scientific knowledge is required for easier management and better efficiency and profit.

3. Availability of desired type of labour is difficult, because there should be some degree of experience for those handling and attending animals.

4. For establishing dairy farm there is requirement for large area of land and larger capital for constructing sheds and

for other accessories. Also there is high rate of depreciation for animal sheds and equipment resulting high cost of maintenance. Moreover recurring expenditure required for feed and labour is quite high making altogether a costly affair.

5. It is not easy to get desired type of dairy animals, hence most often we may have to purchase young ones and rear them to adult hood. Selection and purchase of animals should be very careful and under adequate technical supervision. Also it is very difficult to get good quality feeding materials.

6. Risk involved in the business is more. Dairy animal especially high yielders under intensive management are prone to many diseases, which can be fatal unless preventive and control measures are adopted. Good health of animals is a must for profitable dairying.

7. Milk is a highly perishable commodity and has to be produced under utmost care, further has to be disposed within few hours. Any delay in disposal either due to transportation delay or labour availability cause spoilage. Otherwise there should be facility for processing or chilling immediately after milking.

8. Dairy farming is not a flexible business. The capital once invested it cannot be diverted easily for other purposes. The farm has to be run for many years to make a fair return for the capital which has been invested already.

Types of Dairy Farming

Dairy farms can be classified in to different types based on intensity (proportion of income contributed), ownership and intensity and ownership together. Based on intensity dairy farms can be

Specialised Farms

Farming involves dairying alone or 100 % of the income is from dairying.

Mixed Farms

Here dairying is integrated with other type of farming and dairying alone contribute between 10 and 50 % of the total income and crop production or other farming provides more than 50 % of the income.

Diversified Farms

Here farming involves different activities and income from any of the items does not exceed 50 %.

Based on ownership dairying can be :

Individually owned

Owned by any one individual

Co-operative Dairy

Owned by a group of people as a co operative society

Government Farms

Ownership lies with government either local or central

Collective

Here ownership is a mixture of more than one of the above

Based on intensity and ownership dairy farms can be five types:

Family Cow

One or two cows are reared in the family and mostly family labour is utilized for the same. This type of farming allows effective utilization of house hold resources and meets household purposes besides providing some income through the sale of milk. This is the most popular type of dairying in Kerala.

Part Time Dairying

Dairying is taken up as a part time business along with other primary occupations. This allows earning extra income and utilization of leisure time effectively. In this case also few animals are often reared and usually there will be involvement of more than one person to manage the routine activities.

Commercial Dairying

Large dairy farms comes under this category. Dairying is considered as an industry to produce large amount of milk through rearing of large number of cows. Large farms require fodder production, regular supply of other feeding materials and large quantum of labour. Profit depends upon optimum management.

Coral Dairying

This is the system of rearing only milch cows. Cows are purchased during early lactation and are reared. At the end of lactation they are sold to replace with new ones. This system is practiced in cities where there is high demand for milk. Sold cows are bred at villages and maintained till parturition or used for meat purpose

Milk Colonies

This is advised for meeting the requirement of larger cities, where in cows are reared at some convenient places outside the city. Government usually provides infrastructure facilities for forming colonies and for residing of cow owners. This enables to maintain cities cleaner and ensures availability of fodder and other resources for rearing the cows. E.g., Aarey milk colony (Bombay) and Madhavaram milk colony (Chennai).

Chapter 2
MANAGEMENT OF DAIRY COWS

Establishment of a Dairy Farm

While planning to establish a dairy farm, as in the case of many other industries or business a situational analysis/survey has to carried out as the initial step. This helps to understand the marketing facilities for milk and suitability of the place with regard to convenience and resource availability. This is also important to decide on size of the farm or number of animals to be reared. Nature of demand across seasons, milk requirement, and average productivity of animals to be reared is helpful in deciding the size of farm. More over at least 20 - 25 % animals has to be included extra to ensure required number of milch animals round the year.

Availability of sufficient land suitable for constructing buildings and fodder production has to be ensured. Area required for fodder cultivation can be arrived based on irrigation facilities and type of fodder going to be cultivated. Crossbred cows on an average requires 30 kg green grass per day making around 10 tonnes per year. At this level of consumption, 1 acre of irrigated land or 2 acres of non-irrigated land will be required for cultivating fodder for every 4 -5 cows. Fodder requirement for the young stock also has to be taken into account before deciding farm size. If dairying is taken up as means of self-employment, number of animals that can be maintained with available labour has to be considered in deciding farm size along with other points already mentioned.

Locality

For locating the farm in urban areas, availability of land and feeding materials will be the major constraint, while marketing of milk will be easier and price also will be better. But the best location will be rural areas wherein these inconveniences are avoided except for the need for transporting milk to near by town or demand centres. In villages labour and other resources will be cheaper, avoids problems of waste disposal and environmental problems.

For constructing farm buildings like cattle sheds and other accessories, facilities like access to road, water supply, drainage, electricity, scope for expansion and routine operational conveniences has to be considered. Proper drainage is very important to maintain hygiene and to minimise the incidence of diseases. Lay out of the farm should be such that there is maximum operational convenience, easy access from owners residence, better supervision, less climatic stress on animals and healthy atmosphere. Different types of sheds and their size can be decided based on the number of animals going to be reared and based on scientific recommendations.

Purchase of Cows

Extreme care has to be taken starting from the beginning of activities for establishing a dairy unit. In order to ensure better performance, cows have to be selected carefully and managed scientifically. It is preferable to purchase cows from known sources and near by places in order to avoid the chances of cheating and adaptability problems. Rearing of high yielding cows will be more economic provided sufficient and continuous availability of essential resources are ensured. It is better to purchase cows at early lactation or during late pregnancy and cows of first to third calving are preferred. Stage of lactation can be assessed based on age of the calf, and reliable records if available. Wherever possible attending one or two days at milking will be useful to assess the actual milk yield. Reasons for selling of the cow also may be asked for.

Price of cow is usually assessed based on the milk yield at peak of lactation. In most of the areas rate is fixed as Rs 1000 per every litre of daily yield but this can vary depending upon so many factors. Before taking home the cow, usual management, feeding and health care practices has to be enquired in order to avoid sudden variation.

Transportation can be carried out by walk if distance is short. Transporting by vehicles has to be resorted to if distance is more than 3-4 Kilometres. Whichever may be the mode, transportation has to be done in the evening or morning hours to minimise stress and resultant reduction in milk yield. If the cow is pregnant extreme care should be taken at transportation. It is better to avoid to transportation during very advanced stages of pregnancy. Once brought home the cow has to be housed comfortably and sudden changes in management has to be avoided. Calf if present can be housed in the vicinity in order to avoid excitement and bellowing. If animals are purchased for a dairy farm, introduction of the new animals to the existing herd has to be done after sufficient quarantine period (isolation) especially if the animals are brought from a distant place.

Care of Lactating Cows

Expression of inherited capacity for milk production depends on suitability of environment and adequacy of management. Dairy animals have high metabolic rate and are highly prone to stress. Hence housing should be comfortable protecting from extremes of climatic adversities. Cows perform well in temperate or cold climate and high temperature adversely affects milk production and reproductive performance. Intensive or semi intensive system of management is more suitable and conventional cattle barns are often used for housing.

Feeding

Dairy cows has to be fed according to the level of production and physiological status. Being ruminants they can effectively utilise roughage, but in order to ensure high levels of production availability of sufficient nutrients like energy, proteins and minerals have to be ensured. This can be achieved through incorporation of concentrates in the ration. Ration should contain adequate proportion of roughage and concentrate. Sufficient quantity of wholesome water has to be made available either continuously or at frequent intervals. Actual requirement of water and other nutrients are decided by level of production, body size, reproductive status, climate and so on.

Concentrate in the ration should not exceed 1/3 of total quantity. Ideally the ration for ruminants should provide roughly 2/3 of the

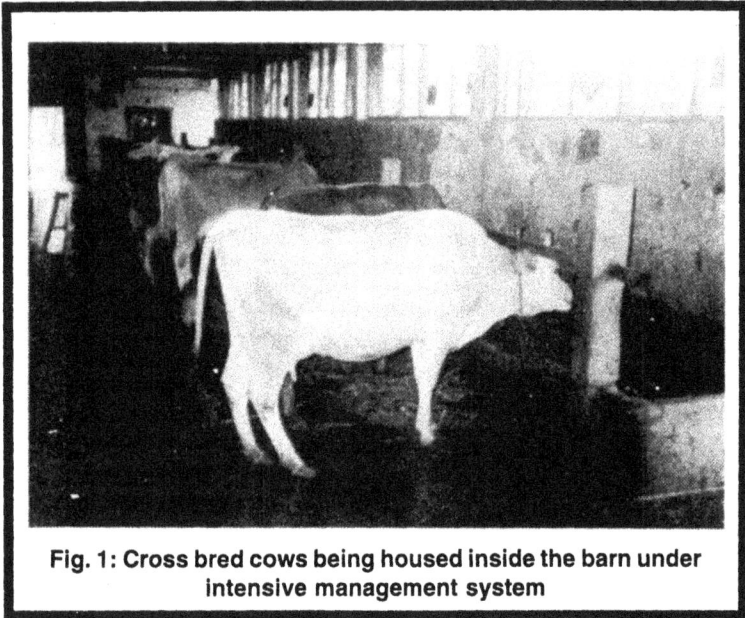

Fig. 1: Cross bred cows being housed inside the barn under intensive management system

nutrients required through roughage and remaining 1/3 as concentrate. Crossbred cow weighing 250 - 350 Kgs requires 25 to 30 Kgs of green grass daily. If good quality leguminous fodder is available, quantity of green grass can be reduced to 20 - 25 kgs with legume and grass at 1:2 proportion. If sufficient green grass is not available preserved fodder like silage or hay can be fed, and daily requirements are as follows:

1. Silage: 20-25 Kgs
2. Hay: 15-20 Kgs
3. Straw: 3-5 Kgs

Along with straw at least 1- 2 Kgs of green grass has to be given in order to meet the requirement of vitamins especially Vit. A. If animal is let out daily for grazing, requirement of roughage can be reduced depending upon the grazing time allowed and nature and quality of pasture. Allocation of concentrate has to be decided based on type of fodder, milk production level and physiological status like growth, pregnancy, work and so on. General guideline for allocation of concentrate feed is as follows:

Table 4

Sl. No	Allowance	Quantity	Remarks
1	Maintenance	0.5 - 1 Kg	Not needed if fodder quality is good
2	Growth	1 Kg	Needed up to 2nd calving
3	Milk Production	1 Kg per every 3 Kgs of Milk	Consider milk composition also
4	Pregnancy	1 Kg	From 4th month of pregnancy onwards

Concentrate feed mixtures can be computed at the farm or purchased from the market depending upon the feasibility and other practical aspects. If purchased, pellets are preferred over mash since pellets avoids selection at feeding, and possibility of adulteration. Daily allocation of concentrate can be fed over few instalments for better utilisation. Mashes should not be fed during milking time in order to avoid feed particles entering the milk. Also moistening of mashes before feeding helps to reduce respiratory problems.

Milking

It is the process of collecting milk from the mammary glands of lactating animals. Milk being major return from dairy animals, timely and scientific milking procedures are very important in order to maintain better production and to make it more economic. Dairy cows has to be milked twice or thrice every day. Usually first milking is done at early morning considering the marketing convenience. Subsequent milking times should be adjusted to get sufficient time interval between each milking. For better results, milker should have sufficient experience and frequent change of milker should be avoided. Milking has to be done under clean surroundings preferably in milking parlours. Before milking, dung and dirt from the hind quarter of the cow as well as the floor has to be removed. Udder and adjoining skin is then washed and then dried by mopping with a towel. Measures for clean milk production has to be strictly adhered to in order to ensure milk of better quality.

Lactation and its Characteristics

Lactation is the stage of mammary function producing milk initiated and maintained by the action of various hormones.

Secretory capacity of mammary gland varies depending upon so many factors such as breed, genetic potential of the individual, stage of lactation, type of feed and other management factors, climate, stress, pathological alteration of the gland and so on.

Standard lactation period recommended for economic milk production is 305 days, including five days of colostrum and 300 days of normal milk secretion. Logic behind this is that under optimum management, most of the lactating animals show heat signs by about 40 - 60 days of lactation, and many of them conceive by 60 days. In those animals milking has to be stopped at 300 days in order to ensure around 60 days of dry period. Also as lactation advances milk yield goes on decreasing and beyond certain point of time production becomes uneconomic. Even though this point varies depending upon so many factors, in majority of the animals it is 305 days. Hence standard lactation period is taken as 305 days for all the animals, but can be extended if conception is delayed.

Lactation Curve

After calving mammary secretion increases rapidly from 0 day to reach the maximum at around 35 days. There after the yield remains more or less steady for about 1 month and gradually decreases. The period of maximum milk yield during lactation is called period of peak yield, which is reached usually between 30-40 days. Peak yield indicates the maximum productivity of that animal and this level can be used to understand the lactation yield of that animal especially while purchasing the cow.

In order to understand the pattern of lactation of an animal, a curve is plotted taking quantity of yield in Y axis and days of lactation in the X axis and is called as lactation curve. The plotting is done based on a day's yield at regular intervals during the entire lactation period and is useful for comparing the characteristics of lactation like persistency. Shape of lactation curve shows minor variation between animals and between different lactation of same animal depending upon of the type of management.

Persistency of lactation means the ability of an animal to maintain more or less same level of yield during a major portion of lactation. Persistency is a major economic character as it determines the ability of that animal to maintain a high level of production over long period during lactation, thus affecting total lactation yield.

This trait is genetically determined even though there is much influence of management as well and often forms a major criterion for selecting animals. Across successive lactation, peak yield and total lactation yield increases up to third lactation, remain steady for another one or two lactation and declines thereafter. Hence maximum productivity of an animal can be obtained during its 3rd and 4th lactation which also has to be born in mind for selection of animals.

Lactation Disorders

During lactation there can occur some structural or functional disturbances which can be either physiological or pathological. Some of the common disorders includes:

Teat Cracks and Sore Teat

Horizontal cracks appears on the teat with exposure of row tissues either on one or more teat. Sore teat is another condition wherein small pustules appear on the teat, which bursts at milking. Both conditions causes pain and some time bleeding as well during milking and interferes milking process. Bacteriological quality of milk also will be affected. Application of lubricants during milking, teat dipping and dressing with antiseptics facilitates healing of the condition.

Hard Milker

Some of the animals are very hard to milk due to tightness of sphincter muscles around streak canal. This in turn leads to fatigue of milker and often incomplete milking. Such animals are designated as "hard milkers". In most of the animals it is genetically determined and in such cases all the four teats will be affected, while in some others it occurs due to chronic infection of teat. In both cases it is difficult to recover and culling of such animals are recommended.

Leaky Teat

In some animals sphincter muscles will be very loose so that leakage of milk either continuously or after letting down occurs. such animals are called as "leaky teat animals". This condition can also be genetic or result of injuries to teat. Animals with leaky teat are highly prone to develop mastitis and bacteriological quality of milk also will be poor. Correction of some cases can be done surgically, otherwise such animals has to be culled.

Swelling of Udder

This occurs immediately before or after parturition due to the influence of certain hormones. Mammary gland, teat and surrounding areas will become enlarged often with pain, warmth and redness. Secretion will be normal and will get cured normally even without any treatment. Palliative measures like spraying cold water and application of demulscents are recommended.

Teat Obstruction

It is a serious condition occurring during lactation, wherein there will be blockage of one or more teat. Often it is a consequence of unscientific milking procedures like thumbing and some time caused by internal or external injuries to teat. Unless corrected at the earliest there will be stagnation of milk, pain, mastitis and loss of function of the affected quarter. Correction can be done surgically or by treatment of underlying causes.

Mastitis

It is a serious disease affecting mammary gland caused by microbial infections.

Induction of Lactation

Lactation is usually initiated by pregnancy by the hormonal action. However lactation can be induced in non- pregnant animals by administering the same hormones in the specified dose schedule and the process is designated as induction of lactation. This can be used in sterile animals as a remedy to minimise economic loss.

Hormones of pregnancy such as Oestrogen and progesterone are administered for about one week so that there will be development of mammary gland and initiation of lactation as in the case of pregnancy. First few days' secretion will be similar to colostrum and there after milk production continues as long as milking is continued. Quality of milk will be exactly same as that of normal milk and there will be no other functional disturbances to the animal as well. However the induction is less successful in heifers compared to cows even though sterility problem is more in heifers.

Breeding

Cows has to be bred early during the lactation period in order to ensure next calving shortly after the completion of standard lactation period. Lactation length recommended for economic milk production from cattle is 305 days or 10 months. In order to achieve this, the cow should calve within next 2- 3 months so that inter calving interval will be about 1 year. For getting this ideal periodicity, the cow should conceive within 60 -90 days of calving. Considering the fact that conception often requires more than one service (Average 1-3 services per conception as is prevalent among crossbred cattle), cow should be bred at the first heat after calving itself, which will be shown usually around 40-45 days. After 40 days of calving cows should be observed for heat symptoms, which includes

1. Restlessness, bellowing, and disinterest in feeding.
2. Lactating animals will have reduction of milk yield.
3. Frequent urination and standing with tail head raised.
4. Running in search of males and association with males if available.
5. Homosexual behaviour (Mounting on other animals or allowing other animals to mount).
6. *Flehmen reaction*: (Tasting urine of other animals and exposing the gum in a typical way).
7. Swelling of the vulval lips and reddening of the genital mucous membrane
8. Flowing of thick, transparent and clear mucous f om the genitalia.

All the cows need not exhibit all the above heat signs, but there will be considerable variation between animals and mucous discharge is considered as the most important sign of heat. In high yielding cows first heat will be prolonged few weeks to few months and adequate nutrition is a crucial factor in deciding the occurrence of heat in lactating cows. There is a belief among farmers that conception during early lactation affects the milk yield so that farmers often wait few months before breeding their cows. This is evident in case of local cows and also in case of cross- bred cows subjected to under nutrition. However economic milk production demands breeding during the first heat itself. Also conception chance is more during earlier cycles and decreases with advancement of lactation period.

Artificial insemination has gained popularity in Kerala than in any other states for breeding of dairy cattle. Accurate detection of heat is an important factor determining the success of artificial breeding. Cow should be carefully observed for heat signs and bred without further delay when heat signs are maximum. Failure of conception is indicated by occurrence of heat signs again after 18-22 days and if so breeding has to be repeated. If no heat signs are shown even after 40 days of breeding, the animal should be subjected to pregnancy verification after 45-60 days of breeding so as to make necessary management alterations.

Dry Non-pregnant Cows

Ideally dairy herds should not have dry non-pregnant cows, and those coming under this category has to be culled and disposed at the earliest. Prompt culling of all those cows not conceiving with repeated service and even after treatments enables remaining cows to be pregnant at drying from milk. Proportion of culled animals in a herd should not exceed 2-5 % and this proportion can be regulated through timely disposal.

Management of dry non- pregnant animals can be done as in the case of growing stock but giving just maintenance ration alone. There is no meaning in breeding such animals towards drying, since even if they conceive at this stage, result very long dry period and economic loss. However lactation can be prolonged as long as there is good yield enabling economic milk production from those nimals. In such case concentrate has to be fed according to the milk yield. Also wherever feasible induction of lactation can also be tried in case of high yielding animals with breeding problems.

Summer Management of Dairy Cows

Lactating cows especially high yielders have high metabolic rate and are highly prone to stress out of extreme climatic conditions especially high temperature and relative humidity. For the same reason dairy cows perform better in temperate climatic regions. In tropical climate cows perform better during colder seasons and extreme temperature of summer causes stress and lowering of milk production.

Heat exchange through skin is poorer in cattle due to very few sweat glands when compared to many other animals. Also crossbred cows have poor heat dissipating mechanism compared to local cattle. Hence high yielding cows shows panting and disinterest in feed along with rise of ambient temperature beyond 30 degree centigrade especially when the humidity is more. This in turn affects milk production through reduced feed intake and other stress adjusting mechanisms in the body. Hence dairy cows should be given special management during summer in order to minimise stress and recommended measures include

1. Plant trees around sheds so as to get shade over the buildings.
2. Height of the sheds should be increased to have better air current inside the sheds.
3. Roofing material should be of less heat absorbing type
4. Walls and roof of the sheds should be painted white and if possible on the top as well.
5. Provide false roofing below the roof using materials of minimum thermal conductivity.
6. Provide air conditioners, air coolers or fans if possible and affordable.
7. Frequent spraying of water over the animals during daytime.
8. Avoid grazing or exercise during daytime when sun is hot.
9. Offer major quantity of feed during night hours or late evening
10. Offer cold drinking water and preferably ad libitum.

Management of Pregnant cows

Once pregnancy is diagnosed, certain alterations in management has to be made especially from the 4th month onwards. Gestation period of cattle is 270- 290 days comprising 3 trimesters of 3 months each. Of these special care is needed during the last two trimesters since foetal growth and associated changes are maximum during this stage. Pregnant animals have to be properly identified in order to avoid repeated heat detection and re-breeding especially in farms. Important care needed during second trimester of pregnancy is nutritional increment for the growth of foetus along with allowance for milk production and maintenance.

Pregnant cows can be housed separately at least from the third trimester of pregnancy. This is to facilitate special attention and minimise stress and other disturbances. Sheds for pregnant cows should be comfortable with non-slippery floors, more space and better water availability. Adequate exercise has to be provided by letting loose into paddocks for sometime everyday, in order to maintain the animal healthy and to prevent overgrowth of hooves.

Drying of Milk

Milking has to stopped in order to get at least 6-8 weeks of dry period. This is needed to minimise exhaustion of body reserves and to form additional reserves for coming lactation. Drying is difficult in high yielders and the same has to be carried out carefully, since improper drying leads to mastitis and spoilage of milk production capacity of udder.

Drying can be done adopting various methods like:

1. *Concentrate reduction:* Stoppage of concentrate allowance for milk production causes gradual reduction of milk yield.

2. *Intermittent milking:* Here regular milking is discontinued so that milk accumulates in the udder and causes reduction of secretion due to persistence of back pressure inside the udder. Excessive accumulation is relieved by intermittent milking at increasing intervals.

3. *Incomplete milking:* Here milking is carried out at regular timings but without complete removal, so that there will be accumulation of milk and drying. But this method predisposes to mastitis than other two methods, hence not advisable.

It is better to vaccinate pregnant cows against major infectious diseases, to ensure protection of newborn calf against these diseases. Also deworming has to be carried out once or twice during last two months of pregnancy in order to avoid infestation of calf within uterus or immediately after birth. At least 2 weeks prior to expected date of parturition cows have to be housed in sheds intended for calving preferably calving boxes. Calving boxes should have non-slippery floors with minimum slope and adlibitum water supply. Calving box provides freedom to move around and calm atmosphere for calving. Feeding of roughage has to be done in many instalments and ration should be mild laxative especially towards end of gestation incorporating more fibrous ingredients.

Signs of Approaching Parturition

As the gestation approaches term, there will be enlargement of udder, progressive relaxation of pelvic ligaments, raising of tail head, swelling of vulval lips and intermittent vaginal discharge of thick and sticky mucous. Engorgement of teats occurs 24 - 48 hours before parturition and abdominal distension reduces 12 - 24 hours prior to calving. Lack of interest in feed, restlessness and signs of discomfort indicate initiation of parturition process.

Parturition process can be explained to take place in three stages. First stage involves onset and intensification of uterine contractions culminating in external appearance of water bag. Duration of first stage varies from 2-8 hours and during this phase there will not be any external changes except signs of abdominal pain. Second stage is rather short (20-90 minutes) and involves breakage of water bags leading to expulsion of fluids and subsequent expulsion of foetus. Expulsion of foetal membranes and onset of uterine involution forms the third phase of parturition and extends from 30 minutes to 6 hours and occasionally even longer.

During the time of parturition preferably the cow should be left free in loose boxes with sufficient bedding and calm atmosphere. Frequent observation with minimum disturbance is essential. Any chance of calving into water channels leading to drowning of calf should be avoided. In about 70-90 % cases forelimbs and head of calf comes out first, while in remaining cases hind limbs leads out first. There will occur some delay at expulsion of head, shoulder region and hip region. If calving is not taking place even after 1-2 hours of active labour or in case of any unusual happening, expert guidance is indicated.

Expulsion of foetal membranes (Placenta) takes place within 6 hours of calving, and if not expelled even after 12 hours manual removal under proper hygiene and care is indicated. Cows will have a tendency to eat the placenta, which may lead to indigestion and decease in milk yield. Hence proper attention is required until its expulsion and removal in order to avoid eating by the same or nearby cows.

During one or two weeks of calving there will be blood mixed discharge from the vagina, which is an indication of uterine involution and is quite normal. During this phase hindquarter of the cow has to be washed frequently in order to avoid attraction of flies and other associated complications. Some of the cows especially heifers will have oedema (enlargement) of udder and surrounding areas, few days before or after calving, which will return to normal after about one week after calving. If oedema is severe, intermittent sprinkling of cold water is recommended.

Milk production and onset of post partum reproductive activity depends upon the adequacy of feeding and other management. Secretion of first 4-5 days is called colostrum, which will be yellowish and thicker in nature, and subsequently normal milk is obtained. Milk yield will be increasing continuously from calving to 30 - 35 days and during this phase concentrate allocation has to be increased frequently in accordance with the milk yield. Also during this phase of rising milk yield some quantity of feed has to be given extra in order facilitate further increase. (This Practice is called challenge feeding). Sudden variations in feed or feeding schedule can lead to indigestion and have to be avoided.

Chapter 3
CARE OF YOUNG STOCK

Care of New Born Calves

Immediately after calving patency of nasal cavity has to be ensured clearing any membranes covering the nostrils and removing the mucous blocking the nasal passage. For this the calf can be lifted holding the hock regions by one or two persons and shaking for few seconds. Sticky mucous if persist sneezing can be stimulated by tickling nasal mucosa using straw or similar flexible things. If there is respiratory difficulty or gasping, respiration can be stimulated by massaging or repeatedly pressing and releasing the chest region imitating the respiratory movements.

Once respiration is established, umbilicus of the calf has to be ligated one inch away from the body using twine or clips. Free end of the umbilical stump has to cut using sterile scissors 1 inch away from the ligated point, followed by application of antiseptics like Tincture Iodine at the cut end. This is to prevent entry of air and accompanying microbes through the umbilicus, leading to establishment of infectious diseases like naval ill or joint ill later on.

If complete weaning is practised cow should not be allowed to lick the calf and the calf has to be removed as early as possible from the vicinity of the cow. Otherwise cow can be allowed to lick the calf to dry up mucous and also to stimulate respiration. In case cow is weak or calf is removed from the cow, body of the calf has to be dried by wiping with dry clothes, gunny bag or straw. This is very important to avoid chilling and also to stimulate muscular activity.

Healthy calves normally stand up, starts walking and suck the udder of dam within 20-30 minutes of birth.

Feeding of Colostrum

Calf has to be fed with colostrum as early as possible after calving. Colostrum is the secretion of first 4-5 days, which is rich in proteins such as globulins (antibodies) and various minerals. Antibodies of colostrum will be absorbed directly from the intestine of calf without any chemical alteration during the first few hours after calving. This direct absorption decreases as time passes. Hence calf has to be allowed or helped to suck colostrum at the earliest and weaned calves have to be fed with colostrum within 0.5 to 1 hour of calving in order to get proper disease resistance.

If calf is hesitant to drink colostrum, it has to be trained for drinking from vessels. This can be easily accomplished by allowing the calf to suck one of our hand finger, and then dip that finger in the vessel containing colostrum so that while sucking the finger colostrum enters into mouth and gains practice of drinking from pail. Colostrum is rich in minerals, which provides laxative property and stimulate motility of gut for passing first faeces (Meconium), which is usually sticky in nature.

Colostrum has to be fed adlibitum during the first one or two days and then the quantity can be limited to 1/10th of the body weight. Required quantity has to be given in many instalments at somewhat regular intervals. Before feeding colostrum should not be heated as it causes clot formation. Excess colostrum can be fed to other calves in smaller quantities along with milk or it can be preserved as fermented colostrum for subsequent feeding. Feeding larger quantities to other calves lead to diarrhoea. Colostrum is highly nutritious and can be used for human consumption also in the form of sweetened products.

If colostrum is not available due to disease or death of cow, artificial colostrum can be prepared and fed to the calf. For this whip an egg in 300 ml of warm water, add half a teaspoonful of castor oil and one teaspoonful of cord liver oil (for vitamin A), then add 500 ml of whole milk, stir well and feed at body temperature. This is sufficient for 1 feeding and similar quantity has to be fed 3-4 times a day. After four days, feeding can be shifted to normal milk as discussed earlier.

Calf has to be properly identified at the earliest, for this commonly adopted methods include tattooing or tagging. Coat colour and markings at this stage are liable to disappear or change subsequently, hence cannot be relied for identification at early age.

Economic dairying necessitates rearing of growing animals for making timely replacement of the herd. Future of any herd depends on how young ones are raised. It is said that 'good animals are raised, not purchased'. Number of young stock raised should be sufficient to allow selection of the best through a satisfactory rate of culling and removal of those with poor performance at various stages of growth.

To achieve satisfactory rate of herd replacement with young ones of breeding age, maximum number of calves has to be produced and reared scientifically with periodic elimination so as to get the best animals for breeding. Since dairy industry focuses mainly on the availability of more number of female calves, male calves can be disposed at an earlier and feasible stage. Also female calves with very low weight at birth or having congenital structural and functional defects can be eliminated from rearing so as to ensure best ones at breeding.

Weaning

Practice of separating young ones from their mother is called weaning. This can be of two types such as complete weaning and partial weaning. Separation of calves from their mother soon after birth is called 'complete weaning' and is practised in most of the dairy farms. Purpose of complete weaning is to avoid the habit of milk letting down by the cow upon sucking by calf, which may necessitate presence and sucking by the calf always in order to have milk let down. This results great management inconveniences especially when large number of cows has to be managed together. Also milking becomes impossible if the calf dies or weaned after the recommended period of milk feeding.

The practice of separating calves after few days or months of suckling is designated as partial weaning and is practised by farmers rearing few cows. Even though calves can be weaned after 3 months of age, following partial weaning, most of the cows will not let down milk properly. This in turn necessitates continued sucking by the calf at least some time at every milking thus prolonging effective weaning age. This reduces total milk yield, makes clean milk production difficult and also affects health of the calf due to its disinterest for taking other feeds and causes other management inconveniences.

Advantages of Weaning
1. No difficulty of milking the cow even if calf dies
2. Correct amount of milk can be given to the calf
3. Actual yield of cow can be recorded and fed accordingly
4. Calves especially males can be culled at an early age
5. Milking without a calf is more hygienic and sanitary

Thus, in those herds with complete weaning practice, elimination of male calves and poor performing female calves can be done without any difficulty at any stage. However in partial weaning cases elimination of poor performers at earlier stages is difficult due to fewer number, sentiments and essentiality for milk letting down until weaning. Weaning is rather difficult in local breeds of cattle as they show very strong motherly instinct, while it is easier in crossbreds or exotic animals. However through early weaning motherly instinct can be controlled.

Weaned male calves can be culled and used for meat purpose either in the form of veal (meat of calves fed with milk alone) or can be fattened for utilisation as tender beef (meat of young cattle). Calves for replacement has to be reared to get faster growth rate and minimum mortality. For this management has to be started even before birth by ensuring better feeding of the mother during pregnancy and proper care at birth so as to get a healthy and active calf. Birth weight is an important factor determining weight gain of calves during early part of its life. Proper cleaning and sanitation, protection from extreme climate, adequate feeding with milk and concentrate feed, timely de-worming and health care are other important things to be cared in order to ensure better growth rate of calves.

Milk Feeding

Milk is more or less complete feed and gives better efficiency than most other foods when properly fed. Calves should get adequate quantity of milk daily according to their body weight in instalments spread over 3 or more feeding times. Complete weaned calves has to be hand fed using artificial nipples or by training to drink from pail. It is better to warm the milk to body temperature for feeding and supplementation with trace minerals deficient in milk. The recommended quantity is as follows:

Table 5

First month	1/10th of body weight
Second month	1/15th of body weight
Third month	1/20th of body weight

For suckled calves availability of similar quantity has to be ensured according to its weight and age. This can be done by periodic assessment of total productivity of mother and accordingly allotting one or two mammary quarters for the calf, or milking out the excess, retaining the quantity required for the calf not milked in the udder and then allowing the calf to suck. In both types of management milk feeding can be stopped completely from fourth month of age onwards.

Required quantity has to be fed freshly, hygienically, in few instalments and preferably at regular timings. Both under feeding and over feeding with milk has to be avoided as both adversely affect weight gain. While under feeding causes inadequate nutrient availability, over feeding predisposes to indigestion, colibacillosis and diarrhoea (calf scour) which in turn leads to weakness, poor growth, dehydration and even death in extreme cases.

Milk Replacer

This is constituted by feed ingredients cheaper than milk and can be substituted for feeding young calves. Replacers resemble milk with respect to broad chemical composition and nutritive value. Replacement of milk with replacers should be gradual to avoid drop in growth rate. It has been found that at the age of 3 months calves are able to consume adequate quantity of carbohydrate and protein through calf starters and good quality green fodder. Complete stoppage of milk feeding can be done at 45 days without any adverse effect on live weight, if they get adequate quantity of replacers.

Feeding Calf Starter

From second week onwards calves can be offered with highly nutritious concentrate mixture called calf starter. Initially the quantum of consumption will be negligible, but it gradually increases and can partially substitute the quantity of milk to be fed and hastens weight gain. Calf starters usually contain high proportion of good quality protein ingredients such as fish meal, since quantity and quality of protein is very important at this stage of rapid growth. An ideal calf starter should have 20 % DCP (digestible crude protein) and 70 % TDN (Total digestible nutrients). Compound feeds containing urea are not recommended at this stage since rumen has not become functional.

ISI standards for a calf starter is as follows:

1.	Moisture (maximum)	10 %
2.	Crude protein	23-26 %
3.	Crude fat (minimum)	4 %
4.	Crude fibre (maximum)	7 %
5.	Total ash (maximum)	5 %
6.	Acid insoluble ash (max)	2.5 %
7.	Common salt (maximum)	1 %

Examples of one calf starter is as follows

1.	Finely ground maize	43 %
2.	Ground nut cake	35 %
3.	Dried fish meal	8 %
4.	Whet bran	12 %
5.	Mineral mixture	2 %

Small quantity of good quality green grass can be given from the first month onwards. From the second month onwards calves will consume reasonable amount of green grass, which will speed up the development of rumen (fore stomach) and its function so that by the end of milk feeding, calf will be fully equipped to digest coarse roughage. Along with increase in the quantity of roughage intake, water intake also increases especially during summer months. Hence adequate supply of clean drinking water also should be ensured in the pens.

Feeding schedule for calves up to the age of 6 months is as follows:

Table 6

Age (in weeks)	Approximate Body Weight (in Kgs)	Milk Requirement (in Kgs)	Calf Starter (grams)	Green Grass (in Kgs)
0-4	25	2.5	Negligible	Negligible
4-6	30	3.0	50-100	Negligible
6-8	35	2.5	100-250	0.5
8-10	40	2.0	250-350	0.75
10-12	45	1.5	350-500	1.0
12-16	55	-	500-750	1.5
16-20	65	-	750-1000	2.0
20-24	75	-	1000-1250	3.0

Other Management

In farms Calves has to be properly identified preferably by tattooing during first week itself. Periodic weighing helps to assess the pattern of weight gain so as to make necessary alterations in management. It is also necessary to compute the correct amount of milk to be fed. If de-horning is practised, that has to done within 15 days of age.

Housing

Calves has to be housed in dry and well ventilated sheds. Protection from extremely high and low temperatures have to be ensured. Properly ventilated individual pens are preferred than group pens or tying with rope or chains. Tying with ropes causes discomfort, abolition of freedom of movement, idling and lack of exercise, while free housing in groups result licking each other leading to hair loss and formation of hair balls in the gut. Damp atmosphere and moist floors cause chilling and predisposes to various diseases like pneumonia, coccidiosis and calf scour.

Health Care

Objective of health care measures should be to reduce the mortality rate as low as possible. To maintain vitality proper nutrition,

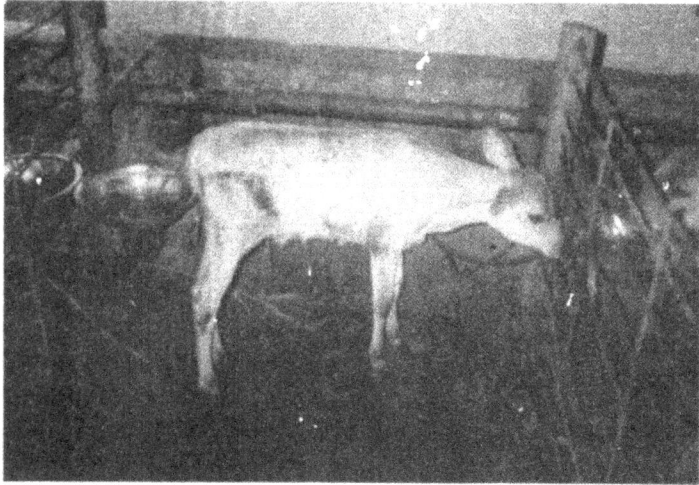

Fig. 2: Calves being housed in loose box

cleanliness and adequate exercise has to be ensured. Supplementation of vitamin A either as injections or in the form of adding fish oil in the milk is recommended in order to avoid its deficiency disorders. Foot and mouth being disease with serious consequences in young calves, vaccination against this can be carried out at fourth month of age. Besides all this signs of any disease has to be attended timely and treated at the earliest so as to minimise its complications. If there is fear of Haemorrhagic septicaemia disease, 30 -40 ml of H.S. serum can be administered at about 15 days.

Deworming

Calves has to be dewormed every month up to the age of 6 months. Drugs commonly used at this age include Piperazine salts, which is mainly targeted against Toxocara worms (large round worms). These worms are expelled naturally by about 4 - 6 months of age, hence Piperazine salts are used for deworming only up to 4th month. From 5th month onwards drugs preferred for deworming are broad-spectrum anthelminthics having wide spectrum of action such as Mebendazole, Albendazole and so on.

Whatever may be the drugs used, adequate dose rate and schedule should be strictly followed. While over dosage causes toxicity, under dosage is ineffective and more over cause development of drug resistance among worms making the drugs ineffective upon future usage even in correct dosage. For best result out of deworming, presence, type of worms and severity of infestation can be assessed by dung sample examination so that effective drugs can be selected and correctly administered. Examination of dung sample is indicated when low weight gain is suspected or when there is frequent digestive disorders.

Dehorning (Disbudding)

It is the process of destroying horn buds at an early age so that growth of horns are prevented. It is done either by using red-hot iron or caustic sticks or electrical dehorner. It has the advantages such as requirement of less space and less danger to man or other animals, while disadvantages include losses such as breed character, style out of horns, and ability to defend themselves.

Best done during first week. Hairs around horn buds are clipped and surrounding areas are protected by applying vaseline. Then rub with caustic potash sticks on the bud for few minutes till it become soft and blood starts oozing out. Electric dehorner is applied after heating to red hot so that horn bud and surrounding skin is burned and later on the bud sloughs off. Both are highly painful and irritating. Hence all necessary precautions may be taken.

Care of Heifers

By 6 months of age calves receiving proper management weigh about 80-100 Kgs with fully developed rumen and are called heifers. The term heifer actually means young female cattle from the age of 6 months to first calving. Proper care and management of heifers are very important as they form the future herd. Better growth rate of heifers enable early maturity and calving so that they become productive earlier increasing total lifetime productivity. For this better feeding and health care are highly essential. However the farmers, since heifers are non-producing and no immediate returns, often neglect them at management.

Heifers can very well utilize different forages to the extent of receiving more than 70% of energy and bulk of the ration. However

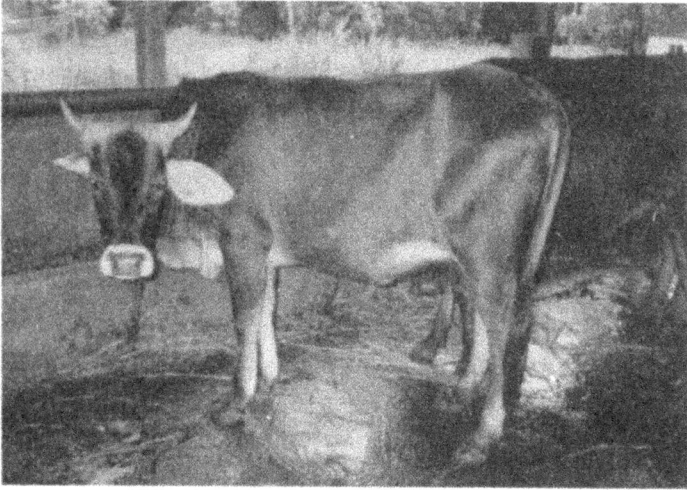

Fig. 3: Heifer being tied up inside the shed
with metal chain

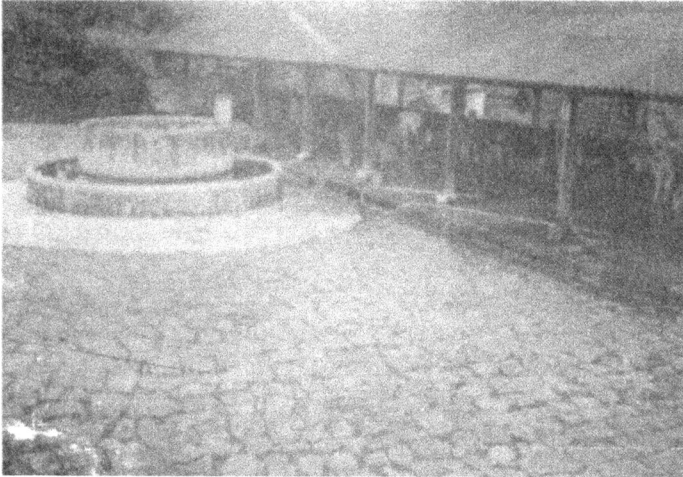

Fig. 4: Model of loose housing system
for growing stock

being the age of rapid growth, requirement of protein is more and protein content of forage will be quite insufficient. Hence to support faster growth about 70 % of the protein has to be supplied through concentrates. However high cost of concentrates often prevents farmers from feeding required quantity and culminates in stunted growth and consequently poor productivity in future.

Concentrate feeds available for adult cows (14 - 16 % DCP and 70 % TDN) can be fed to heifers. If good quality green grass or leguminous fodder is available, heifers do not require concentrates for body maintenance. But a growth allowance of 0.5 to 1 kg of concentrate is required to get faster growth. If fodder available is inferior like straw, an additional allowance of 0.5 to 1 kg has to be given for maintenance also. If proper feeding is ensured, at 1 year of age, heifers weigh about 150 -200 Kgs and at 18 months weight rises to 200 - 300 Kgs.

Over weight of heifers is undesirable and a judicious mixture of concentrate and roughage helps to ensure optimum growth avoiding over fattening. Feed requirement for heifers is as follows:

Table 7

Age in Months	Average Body Weight	Concentrate Feed (Kgs)	Grass (Kgs)
6 - 9	70 -100	1.25 - 1.5	7-10
9 -15	100 - 150	1.5 - 2.0	8- 15
15 - 20	150 - 200	2.0 - 2.25	15 - 20
Above 20	200 - 300	2.25 - 2.5	20 - 25

Concentrate requirement and thus cost of feeding can be minimised by providing leguminous fodder to about 1/3-1/2 of the total roughage requirement or by incorporation of non-protein nitrogenous substances as source of protein. Rumen micro flora utilises nitrogen present in nitrogenous substances like urea and increases the protein availability of the ration in the form of microbial protein. Urea has to be introduced in the ration slowly giving sufficient adaptation period for the rumen flora and energy content of the total ration has to be increased. Feeding of more quantity or introduction without proper adaptation leads to urea toxicity.

For feeding urea, the recommended level is about 1% of the concentrate otherwise required and this much urea can replace about half of the total concentrate required. To illustrate, a hiefer getting 1 Kg concentrate per day can show the same growth rate with 10 gram urea and 0.5 kg of concentrate per day. Before feeding, urea has to be spray dried on to dry fodder like straw or uniformly mixed with other feeding materials. Urea treatment is usually followed for fortification of paddy straw for feeding cattle.

There is great variation in the age for attainment of sexual maturity of heifers. Small dairy breeds can be bred at 15 months while larger ones require about 18 months for exhibiting first heat. Under feeding slows down the growth rate and delays maturity. Cross- bred animals exhibit sexual maturity upon attainment of about 150 - 200 Kgs. Thus faster the growth rate, earlier will be the sexual maturity and increases the productive life of those animals.

Management

Heifers can be managed preferably in semi - intensive or extensive system. Both these systems will ensure adequate exercise and social relationships, which favours earlier attainment of puberty. Houses can be conventional cattle sheds or loose houses. Adequate supply of water and cleanliness has to be ensured to maintain health. Proper identification, Periodic deworming, prevention of ecto-parasites, timely vaccination against major diseases and prompt attention to disease signs are important management measures needed.

Supernumerary teats are seen in many heifers, which are of no functional significance, but affects the appearance of udder and may interferes milking if they are very close to teats. Supernumerary teats can be removed before the heifers attaining puberty. This can be done holding by a forceps and cutting them off. At this stage there will not be much bleeding and quicker healing is effected.

Nose punching, if required for controlling, is done during this period in order to introduce nose rope or nose ring. After proper controlling the heifer, a hole is punched on the nasal septum in front of the septal cartilage using the device - nose punch or any other sharp objects. Piercing through the septal cartilage has to be avoided as the same may cause back ward extension of the hole and delay in healing. Branding if practised for identification purpose is also done in heifers after about 1 year of age.

Health Care

Main measures include Deworming, Vaccination and control of ectoparasites. In order to achieve better health and proper growth rate prevention of diseases are very important. Basic essentiality in health care includes cleanliness and hygiene. Animal has to be washed regularly with thorough scrubbing of the body. In intensive system dung has to be removed frequently and properly disposed Surroundings of the shed also has to be kept clean and dry ensuring proper drainage.

Deworming has to be repeated at least once in every three months. During this age strongyle type worms are more common and are dangerous. It is better to decide the type of drug based on assessment of type and severity of infestation through dung sample testing. Also the quantity of drug has to be according to the body weight. Vaccination has to be carried out against major infectious diseases required as per correct schedule and time. Different types of ectoparasite infestation are common in heifers and use of suitable drugs are indicated based on the type and extend of parasite infestation.

Puberty

Stage of first heat is called puberty. Heifers usually attain puberty when they reach 50 % of adult body weight. Prior to puberty there will be external changes like sudden spurt of body growth and growth of mammary glands and vulval lips. Upon attainment of sufficient body weight for puberty, heifers should be regularly observed for heat signs. During the first heat heifers should not be bred since they will not have attained internal changes required for pregnancy. Stage of attaining ability to conceive is called sexual maturity, which is attained 20-40 days after puberty.

Heat signs in cattle is already described. There will be considerable variation between animals with respect to heat signs and discharge of vaginal mucous is considered as the most important sign of heat. Upon attainment of sexual maturity, heifers should be bred without missing further heat, provided the animal has sufficient body size (at least 1/3 of adult body weight) and good health. Heifers showing poor growth rate, physical defects and physiological disturbances should be eliminated from breeding. This ensures better productivity in their lactation as well as to get healthy progenies with better genetic potential.

Care of Bull Calf

After popularisation of artificial insemination, there is requirement of very little males for breeding purpose. Hence male calves are usually disposed at birth itself or after weaning for meat purpose. Better option will be to rear male calves until fattening and then dispose off at about one year of age. Bull calves are also reared for selecting future breeding bulls or for the production of bullocks through castration.

Male calves can be managed the same way as the female calves during child hood. However after weaning they are fed such a way to get maximum growth rate and to fatten them at the earliest. For this energy and protein content of the ration can be increased even beyond six months with minimum exercise. Castration also hastens fattening. Bull calves for selection of breeding bulls should not be allowed to over fatten and can be managed the same way as that of heifers. Proper screening and culling of poor performers and defective ones has to be done at every step for better results.

Castration

It is the process by which testis of males are made functionless so as to convert bull calves in to bullocks. In cattle, it is usually carried out non- surgically by crushing spermatic cords on both sides of scrotum using an instrument called Burdizzo castrator. For this spermatic cord at the neck of scrotum on one side is brought in between jaws of the castrator and crushed twice at 1 cm apart. The same procedure is repeated on the other side also. On crushing blood supply to the testis are blocked so that testicular tissue degenerates and becomes functionless in due course. Best done at about 1 year of age, since too early or late castration result some harmful consequences. Castration results in loss of male secondary characters of the bull calf and transforms in to bullock.

Chapter 4
HERD IMPROVEMENT

Productivity of the herd has to be improved in order make dairy enterprise more profitable and to meet the growing demand for milk. However milk production being a biological trait regulated by so many factors, enhancement of productivity is not an easy task. Hence there should be continuous effort for the improvement of production potential and productivity of the herd. Production potential of any individual is decided by its genetic make up (Genotype) and expression of the genetic potential is further regulated by interaction with so many environmental factors (Phenotype). Hence for improvement of productivity from the herd, betterment of genetic make up, physical features of the animals and management situations should go side by side.

There are some management techniques to improve current productivity of the herd which includes culling and herd replacement. These processes enable apparent improvement of animals in the herd enabling better productivity. While improvement of genetic potential can be achieved through breeding techniques such as adopting scientific selection of parents and suitable mating systems so as to get desirable characters accumulated in the herd as generation advances. Thus improvement through breeding techniques can be expected only in coming generations, While culling and herd replacement improves current productivity also.

Culling and Herd replacement

Culling means elimination of unproductive or less productive animals from the herd so that the remaining ones produce economically. While herd replacement involves introduction of new animals into the herd to replace those with poor performance.

In any herd there will be animals with different levels of production, age groups, physical and physiological features and disease conditions. When compared to the average productivity of the herd each animal's production will be either above or below the average. For improvement of such a herd we must continuously eliminate those performing below average and replace with animals performing above average so that there will be rapid hike in productivity of the total herd. Here performance does not mean milk production alone but takes into account all other factors indirectly affecting economic production.

Normally about 20% of the animals has to be culled from dairy herds every year for various reasons, Of this infertility alone contribute more than half of the reasons and the remaining reasons are mastitis, old age, major injuries, vices (bad habits) and other diseases. Culling has to be practised in all age groups and some level of culling from growing stock enable elimination of defective animals from becoming future parents. Main criteria for culling at this stage can be growth rate, physical deformities and functional disturbances. To ensure better growing stock for replacement at least 5-10 % of the total number of calves and heifers has to be culled.

Replacement of the herd can be done with animals raised from the same stock or purchased form outside sources. Desirable rate of herd replacement is around 20 % so that 1/5th of the total animals are replaced every year. If young ones are properly cared, more number of animals will be available for replacement every year enabling intense selection for breeding stock. For example in a dairy herd with 100 cows, annually there will be about 80 calving and we can expect roughly 40 female calves. If 10% each of calves and heifers are culled, even after considering about 5 % mortality among young stock, there will be about 30 heifers for replacement, even though only 20 are required per year. So there is scope for intense selection and enables faster herd improvement.

Herd replacement by purchasing animals demands high cost every year. More over it is difficult to get suitable replacement animals in time and even if animals are available, quality of them cannot be ensured always. Also there is lot of difficulties in introducing newly purchased animals in to the herd for reasons such as transportation, requirement of quarantine, adaptability to new management and disease transmission possibilities. However animals introduced from outside sources (out breeding) will enable faster genetic improvement of subsequent generations through introduction of newer genes into the herd.

Vices - means some bad habits of animals, which affect their health, production and management. Some of the vices can be controlled through proper remedial measures, but if no correction is effected through these remedies, such vices form reasons for culling such animals. Some of the common vices in dairy cows and remedial measures are given below:

Table 8

Sl. No	Vice	Remedial meaure
1	Attacking with horns	Dehorning
2	Kicking while handling or milking	Anti cow kicking device, or milk man's rope
3	Sucking its own milk	Anti cow sucking device
4	Withholding milk	Do not frighten or beat during milking
5	Wind sucking	Restrict upward lifting of head
6	Cud dropping	Rasp the teeth to make it even surfaced
7	Hard milker	Congenital - no remedy

Genetic Improvement

Biological characters are determined by genes and genes are carried at least in part from one generation to subsequent ones. Every production oriented character is determined by many genes and interaction of these genes with environmental factors is fundamental to productivity. Even though management enables alteration of environment, manipulation of environment results in better productivity only if the animal possesses genetic potential for high production. Thus first step in production improvement is to enhance the genetic potential, which can be achieved by concentrating and/ or introducing desirable genes into the individual through suitable breeding techniques.

Breeding

The term breeding means management of reproduction through selection of suitable parents and adopting suitable systems of mating so as to get progenies having better genetic make up for higher production. Combinations of genes in the progeny depend upon genes present in both the parents involved. In order to achieve better production potential in the progeny than its mother, newer genes favouring better production has to be incorporated into the progeny by crossing with suitable sires. Thus breeding program should give emphasis to introduce more number of newer genes favouring production through selection of suitable mating partners.

Selection

It is the process of choosing individuals with desirable characters to become parents of future generations. Selection results in concentration of desirable genes for better production. For selection to be effective animal has to be given ideal management so that its genetic potential is expressed to the maximum possible extend. So naturally those performing better will be superior genetically and can be selected to become breeding stock. For selection either a single trait (uni-factorial selection) or more than one trait (multifactorial selection) can be taken at a time. Eg: Milk production alone or Milk production and fat percentage. If more numbers of traits are considered together, selection will become more complicated.

Genes of each individual is contributed from its parents or 50 % each of genes comes from male and female parent. So for achieving best gene combination in the progeny, selection of both male and female parents has to be carried out which is usually designated as male side selection and female side selection. In female side, better performing females are directly selected for breeding based on their milk production or other desirable characters. But male side selection is rather difficult since males do not express milk production trait (sex limited trait). But male side selection is more effective since only few males are to be selected from many individuals and is usually done by indirect selection procedures.

Males are selected based on the production performance of their close relative females to assess their breeding value (production that might have obtained if that bull happened to be a cow). Depending upon the relatives considered selectior can be collateral selection (Horizontal selection), ancestral or pedigree selection (vertical selection) and progeny based selection. In collateral selection bulls are selected based on the performance of their sisters, while in pedigree selection, performance of mother is being taken into consideration.

Progeny Testing

Progeny testing technique of selecting bulls based on their progenies is called progeny testing. Thus, actually producing few of its progenies breeding values of bulls are being assessed. After introduction of artificial insemination and long-term preservation of semen, it is possible to produce millions of progenies from a single bull. In order to test a bull sufficient quantity of semen doses (10,000) are taken from that bull in shortest time possible. The semen is then preserved in liquid nitrogen and the bull is disposed. From the preserved semen around 1000 doses of semen is used to inseminate high producing (elite) cows, so that we can expect 400 progenies including 200 heifers. These heifers are reared until calving and their lactation yield is recorded to assess the breeding value of that bull.

Bulls proved to have superior genetic potential in this way are designated as proven bulls. Only if the bulls are proved superior preserved semen straws are used for breeding, otherwise discarded. The process is very costly and time consuming (taking about 5-8 years to test a bull), but it gives more reliable assessment of breeding value of bulls.

Mating System

Mating system describe the method of selecting mating partners. Mating systems can be classified based on extend of control over mating as well as degree of relationship between mating partners.

Based on extend of control over mating, mating systems can be:

Random mating: Here there is no control over mating so that every individual has an equal opportunity to mate with any other individual of opposite sex.

Controlled mating (non-random mating): Here there is control over choosing partners for mating so that chance of mating for all the individuals are not equal. Partners can be selected based on physical appearance (phenotype) or other criteria

Based on degree of genetic relationship between mating partners, mating systems can be Inbreeding and out-breeding.

Inbreeding involves mating between genetically related individuals (where the degree of relationship is closer than average relationship between any two individuals in the herd). So inbreeding results in accumulation of similar genes and chance of introducing new genes are minimal. Inbreeding favours faster accumulation of certain desirable traits, at the same time there is chance of expressing certain recessive (suppressed) characters in inbred progenies, which is often undesirable. Based on the degree of closeness inbreeding can be further divided into close inbreeding and line breeding. Close inbreeding is between very close relatives such as parent - progeny mating, brother sister mating), while line breeding involves mating between two parent lines such as cousin mating, grand parent progeny mating.

Out breeding involves mating between genetically unrelated individuals (where the degree of relationship is less than average relationship between any two individuals in the herd). This enables introduction of more new genes or variation into the progeny and results better performance. Enhanced productivity of out bred progenies exceeding average productivity of its parents is termed as hybrid vigor or heterosis. Heterosis increases as the genetic relationship between the parents becomes more and more wide or when variability increases. eg: Better stamina of mules than Jack ass or mare.

Out breeding can be four types depending upon the degree of variation or distance of relationship between the mating individuals such as out crossing, cross breeding, grading up and species hybridisation. Out crossing involves mating between two unrelated individuals of the same breed (between two Sahiwal animals), while cross breeding is the crossing between two established breeds (between Sindhi and Sahiwal). In grading up animals of some non - descript breeds are crossed with established breeds in order to up grade the non - descript breed (between Sindhi and local cows of Kerala), and crossing between two species are termed as species hybridisation (between Jack Ass and Mare - Mule, Cattle and Buffalo - Cattalo).

Species hybridisation is unnatural, taking place only with human involvement. Here progenies will show maximum hybrid vigour since parents are totally unrelated, at the same time progenies will be sterile attributable to differences of chromosome number or configuration. (For eg: Mule is sterile as it possess only 63 chromosomes, while the same in Jack Ass is 62 and Mare is 64). Even though Indian cattle (*Bos indicus*) and European cattle (*Bos taurus*) belongs to two species, progenies of crossing between them (Our crossbred cattle) is a fertile progeny of species hybridisation.

Artificial Insemination

Definition

Artificial insemination (A.I.) is the deposition of semen in the female reproductive tract by artificial means. This is most widely accepted tool for breeding most of the farm animals especially cattle. In the natural mating process, the male animal deposits semen in the vagina or other part of female reproductive tract. There are limitations in the number of females that can be mated by a male animal necessitating more males in the population in order ensure timely breeding of entire female stock. This is a great disadvantage especially in those species where productivity is sex limited such as milk production.

Actual requirement of spermatozoa for effecting fertilisation are very few and even if we consider the extra number of sperms required to ensure the situation suitable for fertilisation, maximum number of sperms required will be few millions. But at every mating process the male deposits many millions of sperms in the female tract thus causing wastage of large proportions of germ cells. Through the technique of artificial insemination, semen produced at every mating process is successfully used to breed many females (100 - 500) thus minimising the wastage of male germ cells. Moreover number of males required in the population can be reduced saving huge amounts involved in maintenance of many breeding bulls.

In every species number of males and females taking birth are almost equal. Since AI necessitates only very few males for breeding purpose, intensive selection for the best males is made possible. More over the semen of those best bulls (genetically superior bulls) selected can be used in many females enabling rapid improvement of productivity. Considering this potential of male selection for herd improvement, modern dairy husbandry gives much importance to selection of breeding bulls. Best tool for selection of dairy bulls is considered to be progeny testing, which is made possible by the technique of A.I. Progeny testing necessitates production of hundreds of progenies from a bull in order to test its genetic potential, and is not attainable from methods other than A.I.

A.I. facilitate preservation and transportation of semen to far away places without loosing its biologic properties (fertilisability) so that semen collected from superior bulls at one place can be used at many other places and even across countries without any difficulty so that rapid improvement of animals can be taken up over vast areas in a short period of time. Modern techniques for long term storage of semen enables preservation of semen for many years without affecting fertility so that semen of a bull can be used across many generations even. For all these reasons A.I. is now widely accepted as the breeding tool for dairy animals as well as in many other domestic animals.

History of A.I. goes back to 1322 when an Arab military chief mated a prized mare with the semen of a stallion owned by enemy chief by stealthily collecting semen from the stallion's sheath. The first scientific research in A.I. was conducted by an Italian physiologist namely L. Spallanzani in dogs during 1780. A.I. in farm animals was first successfully under taken by the Russian scientist namely Ivanoff in 1899. In India A.I. technique was introduced by S. kumaran at Mysore palace dairy farm in 1939. Presently the technique is being extensively used for breeding of various species of farms animals and birds and experimentally in other species as well.

Advantages of A.I.

As described above A.I. has got many advantages which are listed below

1. Facilitate intensive selection of male animals for breeding
2. Enables extensive and efficient utilization of superior sires
3. Enables earlier and rapid proving of bulls through progeny testing
4. Saves the cost of maintaining many bulls for natural service purpose
5. Service of superior bulls are made available to many farmers
6. Effectively eliminates diseases transmitted through coitus

7. Semen of superior sires can be used for many years, even after death

8. Animals of unequal size can be bred through A.I. when natural service is difficult

9. Frozen semen technology facilitate import of semen instead of breeding bulls

10. Genetically superior bulls which are disabled or timid can be used through A.I.

11. Facilitate many types of research activities

Besides advantages, there are some limitations as well for A.I. They are:

1. Considerable infrastructure and facilities are needed to establish as an enterprise

2. Well trained operators are required for carrying out the processes involved

3. Infectious diseases may spread extensively if not properly checked

4. Improper selection of animals may adversely affect the improvement efforts

5. Possibility of human errors adversely affecting the fertility of animals

Major processes involved in A.I. are semen collection, processing and storage and insemination. Semen is collected form the bulls trained for the purpose. Usual method of collection involves using an Artificial Vagina (A.V.), which is an artificial device providing similar physical conditions of vagina in a oestrus female such as temperature, pressure and lubrication. Four main parts of A.V. are rubber cilinder, rubber liner, rubber cone and collection vial. A.V. is prepared to get the optimum physical conditions and kept ready prior to semen collection. Then a sexually stimulated bull is allowed to mount another animal and the A.V. is offered so as to ejaculate into the A.V.

Ejaculated semen collected from the A.V. is subjected to various processing. Initially the semen is evaluated for its qualities and poor samples are discarded. Major processing steps include dilution of semen using suitable extenders, packaging and preservation under suitable conditions. Preservation of semen can be done under room temperature, refrigeration or deep freezing. Type of extenders, nature of processing and packaging required are different for each of these types of preservations and storage life also varies with method of preservation adopted. Now a days semen packaged in plastic straws and preserved by deep freezing using liquid nitrogen (-196 °C) is widely used for A.I. in cattle.

Storage in liquid nitrogen is continued without any interruption until the semen is used for insemination. At the time of insemination, preserved semen is taken out of liquid nitrogen so that the semen is brought to room temperature from the frozen state and the process is known as thawing. Thawed semen is loaded in suitable A.I. guns taking all aseptic precautions and is deposited in the female reproductive tract.

Insemination

Usual method of insemination adopted is called recto-vaginal method. In this method left hand of the technician is inserted through the rectum of the animal to locate the cervix of reproductive tract. A.I. gun passes inwards through the vagina is then directed into cervix and the semen is deposited inside the cervix, which is the usual site of insemination. Other method of A.I. is by using speculum (speculum method). In this a glass or metal speculum is used to dilate the vagina so as to visualise the cervical opening and the semen is deposited into the cervix with the help of a pipette. Speculum is not commonly used in cattle now a days, while it the usual method of insemination in the case of small ruminants, wherever A.I. is practised in them.

Insemination of oestrous animal with fertile semen at proper time and using correct technique most often results in pregnancy. However in a proportion of animals pregnancy does not occur for various reasons so that oestrus is repeated after few days. The interval to repeated oestrus will be 18 -21 days in most of the farm animals, corresponding to the duration of one oestrous cycle. However the interval may vary in those animals with functional disturbances. In conceived animals further oestrus will not occur, which are designated as non-returns meaning not returned to oestrus. Such animals have to be checked for pregnancy 2 or 3 months after insemination so as to confirm pregnancy and to make necessary management changes.

Infertility

A temporary loss of fertility (reproducing ability) is termed as infertility while Permanent loss of fertility is called sterility. While sterility cannot be corrected by any means, infertility gets corrected automatically or by adopting suitable treatments. Infertility can be mainly of two types such as anoestrum and repeat breeding. Anoestrum is the failure to exhibit or detect oestrus at the expected time. This is often a consequence of faulty management especially nutritional and correction is by scientific feeding and other management practices.

Repeat breeding means even after repeated breeding successful conception is not taking place. Usually an animal is considered repeat breeder if it is not conceiving by more than two inseminations. Most often it is caused by infection or functional disturbances, which are most often consequences of faulty technique or improper management at some level arising from the part of either technician or farmers or both. Hence for correction besides adequate treatment, improvement of general and technical management is very much important.

Chapter 5
HEALTH CARE

Optimum health is one of the basic requirements for productivity of any animal. Generally health is understood as freedom from disease and discomfort caused out of any physical, mental and social disturbances. Thus health means a state of comfortable living indicated by normal activities and behaviour. In other words health status of an animal can be assessed from various external features and indicators of internal activities. Normally assessment of health status starts with observing the animal from a distance followed by close examination for external features and further based on the examination of clinical samples. External features useful for assessment of health status includes:

General Appearance

Healthy animal will have better physical appearance with well built body, proportionate size of organs, conforming to breed characteristics and with body size comparable to the age of the animal.

Body Condition

Body condition will be good or fair depending upon the physiological status. Bones and ribs should be well covered with muscles and should not be too lean or excessively fat

Skin

Skin should be smooth and pliable with normally grown skin appendages such as hooves, horns and dewclaws. Skin should be free of any injuries or lesions of skin diseases and ectoparasites.

Hair Coat

Hair coat should be uniformly distributed, shining, normal coloured and well grown in accordance with species and breed characteristics.

Eyes

Eyes should be bright and shining without any bulging, discharge or discolouration. Eyelids should close the orbit completely and with adequately grown eyebrows.

Nostrils and Muzzle

Nostrils should be well opened and without any unusual discharge with respect to volume, colour and consistency. Muzzle should be moist and shining, where as in animals with fever or other general diseases muzzle will become dry.

Natural Orifices

There should not be any abnormality of structure or discharges from any of the natural orifices.

Activities

Animal should be alert and active while diseased animal will be droopy and inactive. Healthy animals will show intermittent wagging of tail and earlobes in order to get rid of insects and for heat regulation.

Appetite

Interest in feed is an indication of normal appetite and thus health. Diseased animals will have anorexia (loss or decrease of appetite). Normal acts of prehension, mastication, degglutition and rumination are also important signs of health especially of digestive system.

Posture

Animal should be able to stand normally bearing weight equally on all the four legs. There should not be any difficulty in lying down or getting up. Diseased animals will be recumbent depending upon the type and severity of disease or affections.

Gait

Animal should be able to walk and run normally without any lameness and at adequate speed. Position of head and limbs should be observed in deciding normality of gait.

Excretions and Secretions

Act of passing dung and urine and physical features of these excretions such as quantity, colour, odour, consistency etc should be observed. Similarly secretions like milk, nasal discharge, vaginal mucous, tears and sweat also should seek attention in order to differentiate normal and abnormal features,

Temperament

Behaviour of the animal is important to understand its mental state. Usually animals in heat and those taken to new places will be excited or frightened affecting normal behaviour. Besides that, other deviations in normal behaviour and temperament are indicative of ill health involving pain, irritation or nervous disorders.

Abnormal Acts

Disorders affecting nervous and muscular systems cause various abnormal physical acts (Eg: pawing on the ground, intermittent lying and getting up, circling etc). Continued occurrence of such acts often leads to developments of vices in certain animals.

Production and Reproduction

Maintenance of normal productivity of milk, egg or other products with respect to quality and quantity is an important sign of health since optimum production occurs when all the physical, physiological and environmental factors are congenial. Reproduction being an accessory physiological activity, occurrence of normal reproductive activity forms a comprehensive sign of health especially in the case of females.

Physical Examination

Having observed the animal from distance to understand the fore said external features, next step in the assessment of health is physical examination. Examination usually involves palpation to determine physiological values, besides examination of skin texture, coat condition, rumen motility, condition of mucous membranes and so on. Commonly assessed physiological values include Respiration, Pulse and Body temperature. These parameters are indicative of general physiological status of the animal as they are related to functioning of respiratory and circulatory systems and metabolic activity of the body. These values show slight variations depending upon various physiological factors and environmental variations. However marked variations are indicative of functional disorders.

Respiration

Respiration means functioning of respiratory system and each respiratory movement includes one inspiration and subsequent expiration. Respiratory rate is usually counted based on the rise and fall of abdomen or flank region. Among the physiological values respiratory rate is usually arrived first. The animal is allowed to rest for sometime then respiratory rate is counted for unit of time usually 1 minute. Counting is done from a distance preferably standing at the posterio - lateral aspect of the animal and without causing any disturbance. Besides rise and fall of flank region, movement of the chest, nostrils and air current moving in and out of nasal cavity (observed based on movement of some light materials shown in front of nostrils) can also be used. For better results counting is repeated for 2 or 3 times and average value is taken. Normal physiological values of common domestic animals are shown in table.

Table 9

Species	Respiration	Pulse	Temperature	
			°C	°F
Cattle	25-30	60-90	38.6	101.6
Goat	10-20	70-90	40	104
Sheep	10-20	70-90	39.5	103
Pig	10-20	60-90	38.9	102
Dog	16-30	90-130	38.9	102
Rabbit	32-60	300-330	38.9	102
Chicken	15-20	200-400	41.7	107.1
Man	25	70-72	37	98.6

Respiratory rate is more in case of young animals, excitement, immediately after exercise, high ambient temperature and in diseases involving hyperthermia and affections of respiratory system. Decrease of respiratory rate is not very common though occurs in shock, sedation, certain poisoning and so on. Besides rate of respiration, character of respiration such as depth, regularity, abnormal sounds, abnormal movements etc are also noted so as to get clue to the underlying disease conditions.

Pulse

It is the wave of contraction transmitted from contracting heart through arterial walls. Pulse gives an idea of functional status of heart and circulation and is an important parameter in the assessment of health status. Pulse is usually palpated as contraction and relaxation from peripheral arteries and the usual sites are:

Table 10

Animal	Artery	Site
Cows and buffaloes	Coccygeal artery	Ventral aspect of tail head
Calves, Goats, dogs	Femoral artery	Medial aspect of thigh region

The animal is allowed to rest and the finger is placed at the site with gentle pressure so that pulsation of the artery can be felt. Rate per unit time and other characteristics are noted. Recording of the Pulse has to be done when the animal is under absolute rest and counting of the rate has to be repeated more than one time for accurate results. Pulse rate is more in young animals, pregnancy, excitement, fear, exercise, and in various disease conditions. Interpretation of rate and characteristics will help to assess the health status of the animal.

Body Temperature

It is another important clinical parameter useful in the assessment of health status. In the case of animals rectal temperature is usually recorded using a clinical thermo meter. Mercury column of the thermo meter is brought down (by shaking), bulb of the thermometer is then lubricated and inserted in to the rectum of the animal. The thermometer is then held in an inclined position so that the bulb touches the rectal mucous membrane and is kept for about 1 minute. Thermometer is then taken out, wiped to clean out of dung and the reading is taken. Recording is repeated for accurate results. Body temperature also varies depending upon various physiological states such as young animals, fear, exercise, immediately after food, high ambient temperature and in various disease conditions like fever.

Assessment of health of an animal over a longer period can be done based on the past performances with respect to growth, production and reproduction. Similarly health status of a group of animals over the past can be assessed based on the mean performances of these parameters. Some of the commonly used indicators are growth rate, milk productivity, reproduction rate, birth weight, age of maturity, age of breeding, life span and so on. Growth rate is an important health parameter in the case of growing animals. Depending upon the management conditions growth rate may vary. However under similar management, variations in growth rate is indicative of ill health. Similarly much variations in production and reproduction parameters than expected without much variations in management or environment are also indicative of poor health.

Normal values of life span, birth weight, adult body weight age at puberty, and litter size of common farm animals are given in the table below:

Table 11

Animal	Life Span (years)	Birth Weight (Kg)	Adult Weight (Kg)	Age at Puberty (months)	Litter Size (kg)
Cattle	15 - 25	20 - 35	200 - 800	15 - 20	1
Buffalo	15 - 30	25 - 40	300 - 800	18 - 24	1
Goat	10 - 15	1.5 - 3.5	20 - 60	6 - 12	1-3
Sheep	10 - 15	2- 4	30 - 60	10 - 14	1 - 2
Pig	8 - 12	0.5 - 2	50-150	5 - 8	4 -14
Rabbit	6 -10	25 - 60 grams	2 - 6	4 - 8	3 -15

In clinical set up besides observation of external features and physical examination, detailed investigations are often required for final assessment of health or diagnosis of diseases. This involves examination of clinical samples such as dung, urine, blood, sputum, milk, skin scrapings and semen. These samples are subjected to gross and microscopic inspections, chemical tests and microbiological examination as required for ruling out various disease possibilities.

Judging of Animals

At times it is it may be required to select the best animals out of a group based on health and production as in the case of cattle shows, calf rallies and some other competitions. This process of identifying the best animal is called as judging. Here best animals are decided based upon their external features indicating health and production potential. However in some cases this need not indicate their actual productivity or other economic characteristics. For judging animals are usually classified into different classes based on species (Cattle, Goat, Buffalo), age group (Calf, Heifer, Cow), breed (Cross-bred Jersey, brown-Swiss, HF) and physiological states (Milch, Pregnant).

Usually more than one person evaluates the animal independently and averages of the scores are taken for arriving the final judgement. Judging is also done in more than one round, where in all the animals screened in preliminary round and best few of them are selected for the subsequent rounds. In final round animals are thoroughly screened to select the top rankers. In minor cattle shows score cards are not usually used for judging but judging is done keeping in mind the comparative importance of each of the features.

For judging some guidelines of evaluation are given in sheets called score card. Each animal has to be evaluated in separate sheet. Score card gives maximum marks that can be offered for different body features under four major divisions. Score card for judging dairy cattle giving the details of each divisions are shown below. While judging calves or heifers, instead of dairy characters and mammary system in score card for dairy cows, body size and growth rate in relation to the age forms the major criteria for scoring.

Sample score card

1. *General appearance* (Attractive individuality with feminine vigor, harmonious blending of all parts with impressive style and carriage)

   Perfect score 30

   Breed characters: conforming to the particular breed

   Head: proportionate to the body, large open nostrils, bright eyes, alertly carried ears

   Shoulder blades: Set smoothly and tightly against the body

   Back: straight and strong

   Rump: Long wide and nearly level

Forelimbs: Medium in length, straight, wide apart and squarely placed

Hind limbs: Hock to pastern nearly perpendicular (side view) and straight from rear view

Feet: Short compact and well rounded

Tail head: Set level with back line and free from coarseness

*Tail:*long and slender with well grown long hairs at the tip.

2. *Dairy character* (Evidence of milking ability, angularity, General openness, freedom from coarseness, giving due regard to period of lactation)

Perfect score 20

Skin: Thin, loose and pliable

Neck: long, lean and blending smoothly into shoulders, whither sharp

Ribs: Wide apart, rib bones wide flat and strong

Flank: Deep and refined

Thighs: Wide apart from the rear view

3. *Body capacity* (Relatively large in proportion to the size of the animal providing ample capacity, strength and vigour)

Perfect score 20

Chest: long and deep with wide chest floor

Ribs: widely sprung,

Barrel: strongly supported, depth and with of barrel tending to increase towards the rear

Heart girth: large and deep with well sprung ribs blending into the shoulder

4. *Mammary system* (A strongly attached well balanced capacious udder of fine texture indicating heavy production and a long period of usefulness)

Perfect score 30

Udder: Symmetrical moderately long wide and deep strongly attached showing moderate cleavage between halves, no quartering on sides, soft pliable and well collapsed after milking, quarters evenly balanced

Fore udder: high wide slightly rounded, fairly uniform width from top to floor, and strongly attached

Rear udder: high wide, slightly rounded fairly uniform width from top to floor, and strongly attached

Teats: uniform size, medium sized, cilindrical and squarely placed

Mammary veins: large, long and tortuous

Animal Diseases

Dise ise means deviation from health. Diseases affect the comfort of living and causes decrease in productivity and even death. Thus diseases cause considerable economic loss to the farmers. There are many diseases transmitted among animals and some diseases are transmitted to human beings also, thus affecting health and well being of the owners themselves. Examples include rabies, tuberculosis, brucellosis and some parasitic diseases. Hence prevention and control of animal diseases are of extreme importance, for which exact causation has to be clearly identified.

Animals are susceptible to so many diseases caused by microbes or other reasons. Increased milk production results in lowering of disease resistance mainly because most of the energy is diverted towards production, so that animals are unable to resist disease causes. Thus high production and disease resistance can be considered two sides of same coin so that both sides never comes together. Like that productivity and resistance are inversely related so that when one increases, naturally other has to decrease. This is further facilitated by various causative factors for diseases.

Causative factors for diseases can be of two types such as predisposing factors and exciting factors. Predisposing factors makes the animal susceptible for various disease conditions, while exciting factors initiate the disease process. Major predisposing factors include

Tropical Climate

High temperature along with high relative humidity causes stress to the animal and further stress of high production causes weakening of the defence mechanisms of the body favouring disease occurrence

Poor Management

High production necessitates high standards of management and health care, but farmers maintaining high producing animals often fails to provide adequate management leading to various disease conditions

Poor Feeding

High production necessitates better feeding especially with concentrates, but due to scarcity of feed ingredients and adulteration, quality of feeding is affected making the animal system vulnerable to diseases by toxic adulterants and unbalanced feeding.

Intensification

Scarcity of land and non - availability of pastures, resulted intensification of production and overcrowding. This along with lot of changes in the environment makes the animals prone to many newer diseases or older diseases in more serious forms.

. Major causes for diseases and some of the common examples of diseases are given below:

Developmental Defects

Defects of embryo or subsequent developments affecting a single system or many systems of the body *E.g.,* Cleft pallet, Lameness, Atresia ani.

Physical Injuries

Physical force or energy causes damage to tissues and affects normal living *E.g.,* Accidents, fracture, burns

Functional Disorders

Normal functioning of one or more organs or systems are affected. *E.g.,* Vomition, urinary obstruction, Jaundice

Metabolic Disturbances

Metabolic processes of the body are affected leading to diseases. *E.g.,*Ketosis, Milk fever, Pregnancy toxaemia,

Nutritional Imbalances

Both deficiency or excess of nutrients leads to diseases. *E.g.,* Night blindness, Miller's disease, Acid indigestion.

Climatic Adversities

Extreme climate like high temperature and cold leads to diseases. *E.g.,* Heat stroke, Heat stress, Freeze bite.

Parasitic Infestations

Internal and external parasites produces various diseases. *E.g.,* Maggot wound, Ascariasis, Tape worm infestation

Mirobial Infections

Various categories of micro organisms produces diseases in animals. *E.g.*, Anthrax, FMD, Ring worm.

Poisoning

Different types of toxins causes diseases in animals. *E.g.*, HCN poisoning, Snake bite, Urea poisoning.

Unknown Factors

There are some diseases for which exact causation in not known. *E.g.*, Cancers, Tail necrosis.

Above causes either in single or combination results many types of diseases with varying severity, manifestation and ultimate result. Some of these causes can be avoided through proper and timely management. While for some other reason prevention is not possible.

Based on the extent of tissue involvement diseases can be systemic diseases or local affections. Systemic diseases affects entire body or many systems (*E.g*; Fever) while local affects only one system or part of one system or a organ (*E.g.*, wound). Based on the severity, diseases can be acute, sub acute or chronic in nature. Acute diseases are with severe symptoms, fast occurring and often with serious consequences. *E.g.*, Anthrax, Haemorrhagic septicaemia. While chronic diseases are slow in occurrence, with mild symptoms and long standing. However its consequences vary with duration of disease occurrence. *E.g.*, Johne's disease, Tuberculosis. Sub acute diseases are medium in severity, rapidity and consequences. *E.g.*, Foot and mouth disease, Ephemeral fever.

Generally diseases can be classified based on the causes as follows:

Table 12

Diseases			
Caused by Living Pathogens			
Microbial Infections		*Parasitic Infestations*	
Unicellular	*Multi-cellular*	*Endo Parasites*	*Ecto parasites*
Bacteria	Fungus	Round worms	Flies, Fleas
Virus		Tape worms	Lice, Bugs,
Protozoa		Flukes	Ticks, Mites

Non Living Reasons				
Nutritional	*Metabolic*	*Injuries*	*Toxins*	*Others*
Deficiency, Excess	Disturbances of metabolic processes	Accidents Wounds	Biologic Chemical	Cancers

Basically diseases can be those caused by living pathogens such as microbial infections and parasitic infestations. Disease producing (Pathogenic) microorganisms include unicellular organisms like bacteria, virus and protozoa and multi-cellular organisms like fungus, accordingly diseases can be bacterial, viral, protozoan and fungal diseases. The organism enters the body through various routes of entry and gets established inside or outside the body and produces various disease conditions.

Parasitic diseases belong to two broad categories such as endoparasitism and ecto-parasitism. Endo- parasitism is also called as worm infestation and is usually caused by three classes of worms such as round worms (Nematodes), tapeworms (Cestodes) and flukes (Trematodes). Common ecto-parasites belongs to Arthropoda (Phylum) and can be of two categories such as insects or arachnids. Parasitic insects include flies, fleas, lice, and bugs, while pathogenic arachnids can be ticks or mites.

Diseases caused by non-living causes include nutritional deficiency diseases, diseases of overfeeding, Metabolic diseases, injuries, diseases caused by poisons and diseases of unknown reasons. All diseases seen in animals belong to any one or more of above categories. Identification of the type, causes and mode of transmission of diseases enable early treatment and prevention of subsequent occurrences.

General Measures of Disease Control

Once a disease sign is noticed, the owner or care taker should pay keen attention to detect the progress of symptoms and also to understand the probable causation. Identification of cause of disease and mode of its occurrence is the basic step in controlling any disease incidence. Once the disease or its causation is identified, and if treatment or some management correction is indicated, immediate steps has to be taken up for such treatment or correction so as to avoid further progression of the condition.

If infectious or contagious nature of disease is suspected, the affected animals and preferably in contact animals has to be isolated in order to avoid transmission to other animals. For diseases having long incubation period and possibility of transmission before appearance of symptoms, most of the in contact animals might have contracted the infection. In such cases isolation of all the animals will be difficult and any prophylactic medication if available, should be resorted. If the disease is suspected out of some management problems, immediate corrections in management has to be taken up.

Sanitation has very crucial role in controlling infectious diseases especially by minimising the spread among animals and herds. Houses and utensils should be thoroughly cleaned. Separate utensils should be used for affected animals. Drinking water and other feeding materials should be free from contamination. Flies and other disease transmitting vectors should be controlled using proper methods. Bedding, left over feeds and other wastes of affected animals should be disposed properly, preferably by burning or burying. In case of major infectious diseases, it is better not to use the products during the disease and treatment for the safety of public.

Prevention: Provision of optimum management is very important to ensure better health and strength of natural defence mechanisms so as to prevent diseases. Comfortable housing, balanced nutrition, avoiding sudden changes in feeding, better hygiene, parasite control and other health care measures are very important. For diseases having vaccination prevention can be effected through vaccination in advance. But vaccination should not be carried out when disease symptoms have started.

Chapter 6
COMMON DISEASES

Foot and Mouth Disease (FMD)

It is a commonly occurring viral disease seen in all cloven footed animals such as cattle, buffalo, goat, sheep, pig and even in elephants. Our native animals were much resistant to this disease so that seldom affected by the disease and even if affected symptoms were very mild and less serious. However high producing animals like exotic and crossbred animals are highly susceptible and the disease is much serious in them. Now a days even the wild ruminants are affected by this disease to some extent.

The disease is transmitted mechanically through contaminated water, feeds, utensils and vectors like flies. The disease is caused by different strains of FMD virus, and route of entry usually mouth. Once enter the digestive tract, FMD viruses colonize in rumen, multiples and enters in to the blood circulation. Entry of organisms into the blood is associated with severe fever and subsequently the viruses settles and initiate lesions in tissues of foot and mouth cavity. Hence the disease is called by the name Foot & Mouth disease. Besides these sites lesions are also formed on udder and other parts of the body and in young calves heart muscles are commonly affected..

In affected areas there will be development of vesicles, which breaks of forming open wounds. These wounds becomes infected or infested with maggots leading to further complications. Affected animals will be off feed, milk production drops drastically, there will be salivation and inability to walk. If condition is not attended promptly, turns more serious leading to death even. Pregnant cows will abort and affection of young calves will lead to sudden death without much symptoms.

The lesions have to be dressed with suitable antiseptics and demulscents and fly repellents has to be applied. Proper veterinary care has to be ensured at the earliest to effect control and to minimize complications. Near by animals if infected will take about 3-7 days for the symptoms to appear. To avoid further transmission, affected and in contact animals have to isolated from the herd and treated separately. In some of the animals cured from the disease there will be irreversible drop in milk yield and impairment of thermo-regulation so that animals turn chronic "panters".

Prevention of the disease can be effected through timely vaccination. Vaccination of the entire herd has to be carried out every year. Oil adjuvant vaccine is used now a days which provides about 9 months immunity. Usually vaccination is recommended just before monsoon season since disease occurrence is more during and immediately after the rainy season. Hence vaccination has to be repeated once in every April - May period so as to ensure year round protection.

Rinderpest

It is a severe type of diarrhoeal disease mainly affecting ruminants caused by a virus named as Rinderpest virus. The disease is characterised by high fever, appearance of erosions on oral and rectal mucous membranes followed by severe diarrhoea leading to dehydration, coma and death. The disease mainly affects cattle and buffaloes, while small ruminants are less affected. Transmission of the diseases occurs through direct or indirect contact of the unaffected animals with secretions and excretions of infected animals. Virus present in these materials enters through mucous membranes and multiplies in blood and in lymphoid organs.

Once entered the body, the virus takes about a week to reach peak concentration in blood and this stage is manifested by high fever. Subsequently there will be localisation mainly in alimentary tract and other symptoms start such as anorexia, salivation, lacrimation and appearance of raw ulcers on the oral mucosa. Vesicles are not seen in the mouth as in the case of foot and mouth disease but there will be occurrence of raw ulcers directly.

Lacrimation become more profuse and subsequently purulent as the disease advances. Diarrhoea starts with subsiding of fever and progresses to become more severe and frequent so that animal collapses very shortly and death is very common in affected cases.

Once the symptom starts, no further treatment is effective. Control measures include isolation of affected and suspected animals, thorough disposal of carcasses and incontact materials and proper hygienic measures. Fortunately, due to the intensive efforts for eradication taken up, over last many years the disease has not been reported in the country. Accordingly preventive efforts against this disease such as vaccination are no more recommended and vigilant observation is going on so as to declare the country free of Rinderpest and the disease eradicated.

Haemorrhagic Septicaemia

It is a severe respiratory disease caused by bacteria called *Pasteurella multocida* seen in animals. These organisms normally inhabit respiratory tract of most animals and the disease is predisposed by stress due to conditions like sudden variations in climate. In severe cases there will be sudden onset and symptoms include high temperature, abdominal pain, and respiratory difficulty leading to death in a good proportion of affected animals. In milder form, there will be fever, sudden drop in milk yield, signs of abdominal pain, diarrhoea, respiratory difficulty, oedema of neck and brisket region. Mucous membranes will become bluish coloured and there will be haemorrhages in internal organs.

The disease commonly occurs in cattle during the onset of monsoon seasons. Diagnosis of the condition can be made based on symptoms and also by blood smear examination for the presence of characteristic bipolar staining organisms. The disease can be cured through earlier treatment upon onset of symptoms with suitable antimicrobial drugs in correct dose and schedule. Effective prevention can be done by vaccination. Different types of vaccines are available such as broth vaccine and oil adjuvant vaccine, which has to be administered sufficiently prior to the probable season.

Anthrax

Anthrax is a per acute bacterial disease commonly affecting ruminants caused by the organism namely *Bacillus anthracis* and the disease is more common in some geographical locations. The disease has been reported from different parts of Kerala but not very common now a days. The organism persists for many years in prevalent areas in the form of highly resistant spores and causes the disease upon entry into susceptible animals. Infection is through ingestion, inhalation or through wounds so that the organisms enters the blood through abrasions on mucous membranes and starts multiplication. Animal to animal transmission is not possible, however spread of infection to newer areas occurs through contaminated materials. Human beings are also affected through the handling of contaminated items.

Symptoms start upon accumulation of large number of bacteria in the blood (septicaemia) and in most cases sudden death occurs even before noticing any symptoms of disease. There will be high fever, respiratory difficulty and abdominal pain followed by death. Carcasses will show acute abdominal blot, congestion of mucous membranes and oozing of tarry blood from the natural orifices.

Diagnosis of the condition can be made based on symptoms and confirmation can be made based on blood smear examination for presence of typical anthrax organisms. If anthrax disease is suspected, such carcasses should not be opened either for post mortem examination or other purposes. The disease can be cured through proper treatment in few cases at the first sight of symptoms. Other control measures include proper disposal of carcasses and in contact materials, hygiene and so on. Prevention is effected through annual vaccination in prevalent areas. Inactivated spore vaccine is usually employed which ensures protection beyond 2 weeks after the vaccination.

Black Quarter

Black quarter is a bacterial disease affecting mainly cattle characterised by inflammation of skeletal muscles and subsequent toxaemia leading to death. The organism *Clostridium chauve;* which is an anaerobic bacteria causes the disease and the disease is more prevalent in some areas. The organisms remain as spores in the soil, which are highly resistant and infection occurs through ingestion. Young animals in good health are more commonly affected. Organisms entering blood through mucosal abrasions multiplies in the blood and localises in skeletal muscles especially of the thigh region, hence the disease is also called as "black leg".

Affected animals will show lameness with or without high fever, depression and anorexia. There will be pronounced swelling at the region of affected muscles, with warmth and pain initially and later on becomes cold, painless and crepitating due to gas accumulation. The skin of the affected area becomes discoloured, progressing to dryness and crack formation. Animal becomes progressively weak and dull and death occurs out of toxaemia. Diagnosis based on symptoms and examination of blood smear or fluid from the affected muscles for the presence of typical organisms.

In early cases treatment is effective and prevention can be done by vaccination of the susceptible animals routinely. Different types of vaccines, either in single or in combination with other vaccines are available which ensures adequate protection. Since the occurrence of disease is more during summer and spring, vaccination is advised prior to these periods.

Tuberculosis

It is a chronic bacterial diseases seen in domestic animals caused by the organism *Mycobacterium bovis*. Main routes of infection are inhalation and ingestion and once entered the body, the disease is very slow to set in, hence commonly seen in older animals. Mostly affected sites include respiratory system, mammary gland , bones and nervous system. There will be progressive development of tubercles or small nodules in the affected areas. The disease is of public health importance as it is transmitted from animals to human beings and back, and is of great significance in dairy cattle, due to the possibility of transmission through milk.

In earlier cases the disease will be of no symptoms, except for low production, but the animal will act as source of transmitting the disease agents. The organisms are excreted in exhaled air, sputum, faeces, milk, urine and other bodily discharges. There will be progressive wasting and other symptoms depending upon the organs affected. Even though the disease causes death only in terminal stages, production from the affected animals will be considerably affected. Mastitis due to tuberculosis causes TB organisms to be released through milk and causes easy transmission to calf as well as human beings, unless the milk is properly processed before consumption.

Diagnosis of the condition can be done in early cases based on tuberculin testing so that sub clinical cases can be identified, treated or eliminated depending upon the case. Advanced cases can be diagnosed based on symptoms and bacteriological examination for isolation of the organism or identification of typical tissue lesions. Since long term therapy with different drugs are required, treatment is not advised in the case of farm animals, but early disposal is the recommended practice.

Brucellosis

It is another bacterial disease of dairy animals having public health importance. The disease in large ruminants is caused by the organisms called *Brucella abortus* and is characterised by abortion during late gestation. The organism gains access into the body through contact with mucous membranes and localise mainly in reproductive system and joints. In females organisms multiplying in gravid uterus causes abortion and the organisms are excreted through aborted mass and subsequent discharges, which is infectious to in contact animals and human beings. Males if affected organisms localise in testicles and accessory sex glands and excrete organisms through semen causing infection to some females served subsequently unless the semen is properly disinfected.

In cows abortion of the pregnancy following infection occurs after 5th month. However abortion may not occur in subsequent pregnancies. Affection of reproductive system also leads to infertility in both males and females, while affection of joints cause arthritis and lameness. Human beings coming in contact with infectious material can get the disease with similar manifestations such as affections of uterus, ovaries and testicles leading to reproductive problems, but mostly manifested as undulent fever.

Diagnosis is done based on symptoms and using different serological tests to detect brucella antigens in blood, milk or other discharges. In animals treatment is not usually adopted, instead the affected animals detected at screening tests are promptly culled and disposed. Prevention can be done through hygienic measures and routine vaccination. Brucella strain - 19 vaccine is being used in areas, where the disease is prevalent, on order to protect the animals not affected so far.

Babeciosis

It is a protozoan disease caused by the organisms namely Babesia. It commonly affects cattle and animals of all age groups are affected. The disease is transmitted by ectoparasites such as ticks. The organisms entering the body reach blood wherein they multiply inside red blood cells. There will be high fever followed by passing of red or coffee coloured urine. Multiplication of the organisms leads to breakage of RBC s with release of haemoglobin pigment, which is causing the change in colour of urine. Animal becomes off feed, and in some of the animals especially young ones, there will be diarrhoea along with passing of coffee coloured urine.

The disease requires prompt treatment with suitable anti protozoan drugs. Other wise there will be extensive damage of blood cells and resultant weakness, anaemia, liver damage, jaundice and death. However timely treatment gives immediate recovery even with a single administration of the drugs. Other preventive measures include controlling ticks and other ectoparasites.

Coccidiosis

It is a commonly occurring protozoan disease of calves characterised by blood mixed diarrhoea. The disease is seen in most species of animals and birds and even in adults. The causative organism in cattle belongs to the Genus Eimeria. The disease is caused by ingestion of oocyst of the protozoan in large numbers due to contamination of feed and water. Flies also play a major role in transmitting the oocysts. Organism multiplies in intestinal mucous membrane and its damage leads to bleeding, which progressively increases as the disease continues.

The disease appears as simple diarrhoea later on progressing to dysentry (blood mixed diarrhoea). In advanced cases there will be voiding of blood as such. Animal becomes weak and dehydrated and collapses if the disease continues. Confirmation of the disease can be made through microscopic examination of dung sample and demonstration of coccidial oocysts. Early treatment with suitable anti- coccidial drugs is indicated in order to effect cure and to prevent further spread of the condition to other animals. If the disease is prevalent in an area, prevention of the condition can be made by addition of drugs called coccidiostats in the feed along with proper sanitation and hygiene.

Milk Fever

It is disease seen commonly in dairy cattle and goats during the phases of peak lactation or advanced pregnancy (Also called as parturient paresis). The disease arises due to deficiency of calcium to meet the increased demand of late pregnancy or high milk yield. Usually when the calcium availability through feed becomes deficient, animal system mobilises calcium from the bones with the help of certain hormones. When the availability even from this source become insufficient, there will develop symptoms of hypocalcaemia. Immediate causes for the condition includes actual deficiency of calcium in the feed or presence of excess phosphorus, failure of calcium absorption from the gut and deficiency of parathyroid hormone

Calcium is required for maintenance of muscle tonicity and various other metabolic processes and calcium deficiency is thus manifested mainly as motor paralysis. Affected animal will show weakness, decrease in production and depression. Some animals show transient excitement, muscular shivering, and stiffness of limbs. As the condition progresses, there will be staggering and inability to get up, subsequently leading to recumbency and coma. If the cases are not treated in time, the animal may collapse due to the arrest of respiratory muscles. Affected animal will be lying down in sternal recumbency with the head and neck tilted to one side, however in advanced cases lies down in lateral recumbency.

Diagnosis of the condition can be done based on symptoms and also stage of affection. Treatment involves calcium administration in the form of injection so as to ensure availability of calcium at the earliest. There will be quick response to calcium therapy in most animals especially if the treatment was in time. However few animals will be reluctant to get up and become downer cow. Chance of becoming downer is more in advanced pregnant animals and in such cases inducing abortion is indicated to save the animal. Administration of calcium has to be repeated at suitable intervals and provisions for continuous availability is made through nutritional correction and other means.

Control measures include ensuring proper availability of calcium in the feed and also its proper absorption and availability maintaining proper balance of nutrient, and avoiding digestive tract problems. Proper ratio between calcium and phosphorus has to be maintained in the ration and adequate availability of vitamin D has to be ensured.

Ketosis

The condition is due to impaired metabolism of carbohydrate in the body and the condition is termed as acetonemia in cattle and pregnancy toxaemia in sheep. Glucose is the immediate source of energy and insufficient availability of the same to meet increased energy requirements of certain physiological conditions like pregnancy and high milk production leads to excessive mobilisation of fat. Fatty acid metabolism in turn leads to accumulation of by products namely ketone bodies in the blood, which in turn produces the disease manifestation. Major ketone bodies are acetone and aceto acetic acid and are excreted in urine and other secretions as well.

Affected cows become weak and production goes down drastically. There will be loss of appetite, disinclination to move and wasting. In advanced cases animal become recumbent and sometime there will be muscular shivering and increased sensation. Some animals will show more of nervous symptoms with muscular tremors, shivering, grinding of teeth, intermittent falling and excitement, which is usually referred as nervous form of ketosis and is due to the effect of ketone bodies on the brain. In sheep also symptoms will be more of nervous type and is usually seen in advanced pregnancy especially when there is multiple foetuses or deprivation of feed due to other reasons.

Diagnosis can be made based on the symptoms and stage of occurrence and other circumstances. Treatment involves immediate administration of glucose and ensuring continuous availability through administration of suitable hormones and other gluconeogenic substances orally or systemically. Prevention can be effected to some extent through proper feeding management and ensuring extra allowance during the phases of extra demand. Avoidance of pre disposing factors such as drastic variations in plane of feeding, severe worm infestation, inclement weather and other diseases will be of use in prevention. In goats both forms of disease such as pregnancy toxaemia and acetonemia of lactation have been reported.

Mastitis

Mastitis means inflammation of mammary glands and is usually caused by various types of bacteria, fungi and so on. Organisms gaining entry into the udder through teat or through systemic circulation under favourable conditions multiplies inside the udder tissue causing mastitis. Organisms causing mastitis are most often, normal inhabitants of animal skin or premises such as streptococcus, staphylococcus, corynebacterium and E coli. Udder being rich in milk constituents the organisms entered multiplies rapidly utilising the nutrients and producing various metabolic wastes. In the effort to prevent the microbes there arises tissue reactions, which if prolonged leads to loss of secretory function of the udder tissue.

In acute cases there will be rapid swelling of the udder, pain and warmth and as the condition progresses, udder becomes hard in consistency and secretion will turn abnormal. One or more quarters of the udder might have affected. There will be associated systemic signs such as fever, anorexia and drastic reduction in milk

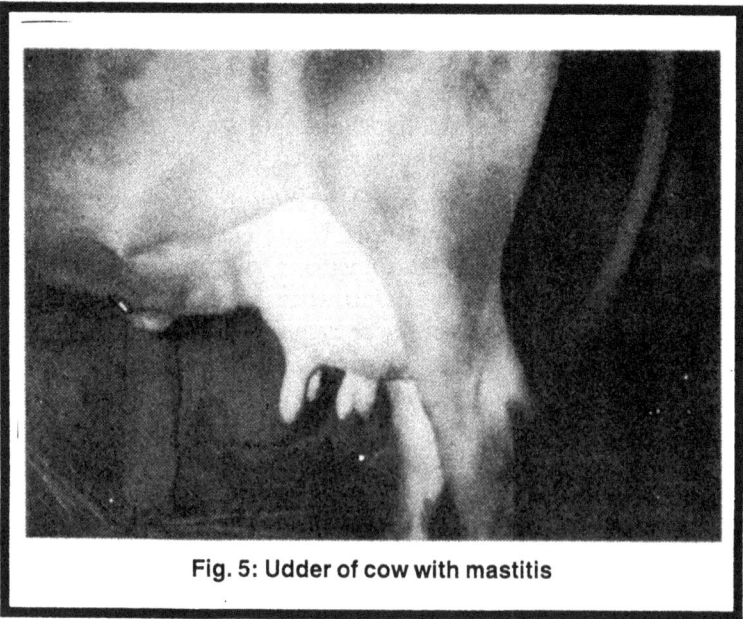

Fig. 5: Udder of cow with mastitis

yield. The condition if not treated promptly leads to toxaemia, recumbency and even death. Also treatment becomes ineffective if there is undue delay so that the secretory tissues become hard and non-functional, which is irreversible. Treatment includes administration of suitable antibiotics along with other supportive therapies.

However in mild cases of mastitis, there will be no detectable clinical signs except for reduction in milk yield. Such cases are termed as sub clinical mastitis. Detection of sub clinical mastitis is done through testing of milk with suitable testing solutions such as California mastitis test reagent. Those detected at this screening are treated suitably so that progression of sub clinical mastitis into clinical cases can be prevented through easier and effective treatment.

Diagnosis of mastitis cases can be done based on symptoms and culturing of milk if possible to identify the causative organisms. Acute cases have to be treated at the earliest in order to minimise further damage to secretory tissues of udder. Prevention of mastitis is done through practices such as teat dipping, hygienic measures, dry cow therapy, and regular screening for sub-clinical cases and prompt treatment. No vaccination is available since the causative organisms are most often opportunistic and variable.

Worm Infestation

It is another chronic disease condition especially seen in young animals and causing considerable economic loss affecting growth and production. Various types of worms infest animals such as round worms, tapeworms and flukes. Round worms are of many types seen in all age groups and is most important. Affected animals will show poor growth, low production, weakness, digestive problems, anaemia, delayed reproduction and so on. This may also pre dispose to various other disease conditions.

Diagnosis of the condition can be made based on symptoms, detection of worms in the dung and screening for ova. Dung sample examination enables detection of ova of worms and thus to assess nature and severity of infestation. Treatment is done administering suitable anthelminthics in correct dose and schedule. Prevention of worm infestation is by periodic deworming. During first 6 months of life deworming is done at 1month interval starting from 15 -20 days. Subsequently the frequency can be reduced to once in three

months up to 18 months and once in 6 months thereafter. During the
first 4 months peperazine salts are recommended for deworming,
while other broad-spectrum anthelminthics or specific drugs as per
indication can be used later on.

Chapter 7
MANAGEMENT OF OTHER DAIRY SPECIES

Besides cows other dairy animals reared in Kerala include buffaloes and goats. Even though management of these animals are not much different from that of cattle, the main differences in care management of these species are described in this chapter

Management of Buffaloes

Buffaloes are the major contributors of milk in India with 54 % of total production contributed by them. Also India holds the largest population of buffaloes in the world amounting to 75 millions forming 54 % of world buffalo population. India has the best milch breeds of buffaloes such as Murrah and Surti, and are well adapted to hot humid and arid regions of the country. While the situation in Kerala is entirely different since milk production contributed by buffaloes are very meagre. There is scarcity of good milch breeds and buffalo population is also very small and rapidly shrinking. According to 1996 census there were only 1.65 lakhs buffaloes only in Kerala forming less than 3 % of total livestock population and from 1987 to 1997 buffalo population reduced to half (-49.8 %) showing a discouraging trend in buffalo production.

Buffaloes are very sturdy and resistant, hence elaborate housing facilities are not an essentiality. Buffaloes are very fond of moist atmosphere such as damp floorings, exposure to rain and wallowing in water. However due to their black colour, their skin absorb more heat energy and are more prone to heat stress. During summer months buffaloes need wallowing in water at least once in a day or intermittent spraying of water on the body to get rid of excess heat. Housing should be such a way providing maximum protection from direct sunlight, excess heat and providing cool atmosphere.

Compared to cattle buffaloes are bigger in size requiring more quantity of nutrients for maintenance. However they can consume and utilise more of (3-4 % of body weight) fibrous feed materials than cattl: hence they can be maintained well with poor quality roughage and less concentrate. Buffaloes require 30-35 Kgs of green grass for maintenance and if quality of grass is good they do not require any concentrate for maintenance. Since buffalo milk is having high proportion of fat and total solids, nutrient requirement for milk production is more and 1 kg of concentrate need to be allowed for every 2.5 litres of milk produced. Other feeding practices are similar to that of cattle.

Under optimum management buffalo heifers attains puberty at 2-2.5 years (300 - 350 Kgs) and can be bred at second or third heat. Heat symptoms are similar to those of cattle with frequent urination more pronounced. Artificial insemination is practised widely but not as successful as that of cattle. Gestation period is about 300 -310 days. After calving reproductive cycle starts by about 90 - 120 days and next calving can be expected by about 15 - 18 months. Most buffaloes show temporary arrest of reproductive activity during extreme summer months and is called as summer sterility.

Buffalo calves are more susceptible to round worm infestation. Hence timely deworming is a must. Same schedule as in the case of cattle can be followed. Vaccination against major infectious diseases is also advised even though buffaloes are more resistant to most diseases than cattle. Buffalo bullocks are used for working since they are very strong and sturdy work animals for farm and road works.

Management of Goats

Goats are reared mainly as dual purpose animals in villages. Total goat population in India comes to 1/5th of the total world population amounting to 110 millions. Most goats in India belongs to dual purpose breeds and are poor milk producers except few dairy breeds such as Jamnapari and Beetal. Hence goats as whole contribute less than 2 % of the total milk production in India. In Kerala goat population at present comes 18 lakhs and over the years there is an increasing trend indicating gaining popularity for goat production. Heavy demand and high price of goat meat are major reasons behind this.

Goats do not require elaborate housing and most commonly a lean to type housing is provided. Semi intensive system of management is widely practised so that significance of housing is only as a night shelter, and are usually termed as cages. Goats require dry atmosphere and are very resistant to high temperature, however goats are easily affected by rain and damp atmosphere. Cages or houses should ensure proper drainage and protection from chilling. Cages should be raised from the ground level and each goat requires roughly 1meter square floor space area inside the cage.

Goats have high rate of basal metabolism and require more energy for maintenance. Goats can consume high proportion of dry matter in the ration (4 - 5 % of body weight) and can efficiently utilise fibrous feed ingredients. Water consumption is comparatively less, and requirement of water for other management purpose is also minimum. For feeding, green grass or tree leaves are the preferred items. If 3-5 Kgs of tree leaves are available as roughage, there is no concentrate requirement for maintenance. But for growth, pregnancy and each Kg of milk produced 300 g of concentrate mixture have to be given. Ready made goat feed if not available cattle feed can be used or suitable feed can be prepared at our own.

Goats have high reproductive rate. Puberty is attained by about 5-8 months. Heat symptoms mainly include inappitence, restlessness, frequent bleating, wagging of tail, search for male, homosexual behaviour, vulval swelling and mucous discharge from vagina. Breeding is usually done naturally and gestation period is 140 - 150 days. Most often there will be more than 1 kids. First kidding takes place by about 10-12 months and subsequent kidding can be expected by every 7-10 months enabling 3 Kidding in every two years.

Standard lactation period is 6 months and colostrum period is 3-4 days. Unlike cattle letting down of milk occurs many times a day in response to kid sucking or milking. Weaning is not usually practised until 3 months. Kids have to be fed with adlibitum colostrum up to 4 days and thereafter milk at roughly 1/5th of birth weight up to 3 months. From second month onwards, small quantity of feed and grass can be offered to kids with gradual increments so that reasonable quantity is consumed by the time of weaning.

Goats are highly resistant to most diseases. Kids have to be dewormed from third month onwards. Ascarid type of worms is not seen in kids but strongyle type worms are common. Deworming has to be repeated every 2-3 months for kids and at every 6 months for adults. Vaccinations against infectious diseases are not usually done but are advised against major disease. Digestive disorders like indigestion and diarrhoea are common in goats, which can be avoided proper nutritional management and timely deworming. Pregnant and lactating does requires nutritional supplementation of essential minerals and vitamins if deficiency is prevalent in that locality.

Chapter 8
MILK PRODUCTION

Milk is the normal secretion of mammary glands and is produced by the female animal in order to nourish its young ones. Hence secretion of milk is initiated during the later part of gestation and is continued till the young one attains nutritional independence or even for some more period. However through human involvement milk production of dairy animals have been increased many times than what is required for nourishing the young one both in respect of volume of daily secretion (daily milk production) and the total length of secretory period (length of lactation). For *e.g.*, While non dairy breed of cows produces milk only to the requirement of their young one (1-3 litres for a period of 3-6 months only), a dairy cow produces up to 20 - 40 litres per day over a period of 300 - 400 days and even more even though the calf's requirement is only 2- 4 litres for 3- 4 months only. Thus physiology of dairy animals has been manipulated to function as a biological machine for producing milk for human interests.

The period of secretion of milk is usually designated as lactation period, which is highly variable between species and between individuals of same species depending upon so many physiological and environmental factors. Major factors include genetic quality of the animals, body size, general health status and especially health of the udder, suitability of the environment especially the climate and management practices, adequacy of nutrition, absence of diseases and so on. Animals getting similar management and environment also show considerable variation in the pattern of milk secretion. During the same lactation period of an animal, volume and composition of milk secreted changes depending upon factors such as stage of lactation, number of lactation, occurrence of pregnancy during the lactation and so on, besides above mentioned factors.

Milk Formation

Milk is formed inside mammary glands, which are modified skin glands (muco-cutaneous glands). Development of primitive udder tissue takes place during embryonic life and after the birth of female animal, growth of udder tissue takes place in different stages At the time of birth there will be presence of small teats, which undergoes a second spurt of growth during pre pubertal stage. Further growth of udder tissue occurs during pregnancy. Udder shows enlargement from the second trimester of pregnancy and is continued for few days after delivery. Maximum growth of udder is occurring during the last month of gestation. These growth phases are caused by the levels of hormones such as oestrogen and progesterone occurring in the body of these animals. For the same reasons if we give these hormones in regulated quantities, growth and function of mammary glands can be induced artificially.

As discussed earlier, udder tissue is formed of numerous ducts, ductules and alveoli. Alveoli are the functional unit of udder tissue and synthesis of milk takes place in these microscopic chambers. Alveolar wall is formed of a single layer of epithelial cells (alveolar epithelial cells), which is surrounded by numerous capillaries, lymphatics and nerve fibres. Spaces between the alveoli are filled with connective tissue and smooth muscle fibres. Also there are numerous, blood vessels like arterioles and venules in addition to ductules and ducts connecting the alveoli to gland cistern - the cavity of each udder. Raw materials for the synthesis of milk inside the alveoli are obtained from the blood flowing through capillaries around each alveoli and the same way by products of synthesis are also removed.

Major components of milk are water and solids like fat, proteins, carbohydrates, minerals and vitamins. Water forms about 87.5 % of milk, which is taken directly from the blood by diffusion, filtration and osmosis through alveolar epithelial cells. Along with water minerals and vitamins present in the milk are also permitted to enter the alveoli. Other macro-compounds such as carbohydrate, fat and protein are synthesised inside alveolar epithelial cells and secreted into the alveoli. Raw materials for these synthetic processes are taken from and the waste products are sent out through the blood. Thus for forming each drop of milk enormous quantity of blood has to flow through the alveolar capillaries. As the secretory capacity of the udder increases there will be proportionate increase in the blood flow through the udder, for the same reason size of milk vein is considered as an important sign of milk production ability of the animal.

Major carbohydrate present in the milk is lactose, which is formed by the union of one molecule each of glucose and galactose. Glucose molecules are taken from the blood and few glucose molecules are converted into galactose and these molecules are then united to get lactose inside the cells. Casein and other milk proteins are synthesised inside the cells through the usual process of protein synthesis. Similarly fat is produced inside the cells either by synthesis using butyric acid present in the blood or by transformation of fat available from the blood. Each of the milk constituents reaches the alveoli in adequate proportion and gets mixed up to form the final secretion called milk. Alveolar epithelial cells mainly control all these processes, even though various hormones and nerve impulses have regulatory roles on it.

Milk Ejection

Milk formed inside the alveoli are retained there for the most parts until the next milk removal. Milk is removed from the udder either by sucking of the young one or by the process of milking. Milk removal is facilitated by the process called milk ejection reflex or letting down reflex. This is a conditioned reflex initiated by certain external stimuli such as sucking the udder by the calf, or washing or milking the udder by the milker etc. In due course of lactation animals get conditioned to more signals like arrival of milking time, sight of milker, sound of milking pails, milking of nearby animals, sound of milking machine operating etc.

Tactile stimuli from the udder or other signals from the surroundings, causes nervous stimulation leading and internal processes leading to release of the hormone called Oxytocin from the endocrine gland - posterior pituitory. Oxytocin released into blood reaches the udder tissue and causes contraction of smooth muscle fibres. This in turn causes shrinkage of alveoli so that milk is pumped out of the alveoli into the ducts and gland cistern and the resultant engorgement of the udder with milk is usually referred to as letting down of milk. Letting down of milk is very important in deciding the easiness of milk removal, volume and composition of milk produced etc.

Hormone oxytocin once released into the blood it has a half-life of about 8 minutes only since it is metabolised rapidly in the blood. More over in the case of exotic and cross bred dairy animals, release of oxytocin (letting down reflex) will occur only once during a milking time. Practical implication of this is that milking process has to be done as quickly as possible once the milk is letdown. Oxytocin once disappears from the blood, smooth muscle fibres relaxes and alveoli expands back into their original size. This in turn not only suspends further release of milk, but draws back the milk already released into the ducts and cistern thus affecting the quantity of milk yield. Hence even in the case of high yielding animals milking has to be completed within 8 minutes. However in the case of local cows and goats more than one letting down is common during each milking time.

Oxytocin in the blood is also neutralised by another hormone released from the adrenal gland. Adrenalin is secreted by adrenal gland and released during circumstances leading to pain, fear, anger etc, which act as a biological neutraliser of oxytocin. Hence inflicting pain like beating, rough handling etc and frightening or disturbing the animal by loud noise, unusual places, strangers, change of milkers, change of milking time, loss of calf etc affect milk yield by hastening disappearance of oxytocin and interfering letting down of milk. Hence such circumstances have to be avoided to the possible extent and milking animals has to be treated well in order to enhance milk yield out of them.

Milk Removal

Milk produced inside the mammary gland is normally removed by either of the two processes such as sucking by the young one or milking. In both these processes, milk stored in the gland cistern and teat cistern are driven out of the udder tissue through pressure changes created on the outer surface of teat. The letting down of milk occurs just before milk removal so that teat cistern and gland cistern gets engorged with milk. This in turn increases the pressure difference between inside and outside of udder tissue facilitating easy milk removal through application of either negative or positive pressure on the teat. Milk released into the teat cistern is retained there by tight closure of streak canal by its surrounding sphincter muscles, preventing free flowing out of milk. However in some of the animal following letting down there will be free flow of milk due to weak sphincter muscles and the pressure rise consequent to letting down of milk (leaky teat).

Milk is secreted originally to suckle the calf and is the most natural way of milk removal. The mechanism here is application of both negative and positive pressure of the teat. The calf takes the teat into the mouth and upper part of the teat is firmly locked in between the lower incisors and dental pad and then the head is pulled down ward or sideways. By this process milk got trapped within the teat cistern is forced out of the teat due to the squeezing action of incisors and dental pad (positive pressure). Simultaneously negative pressure is also applied near the streak canal to make the process more effective. For this mouth opening with the teat is tightly closed by apposition of both upper and lower lips. Then tongue is positioned first to fill entire mouth cavity, followed by slow pulling backwards. Tongue thus functions similar to piston of a syringe and negative pressure is created inside the mouth cavity, which in turn pulls milk out of the teat along with the squeezing action mentioned earlier.

Milking

This term generally denotes the removal of milk from udder with involvement of human activity. Purpose of milk extraction can be for human consumption or feeding young animal itself as in the case of weaning. Depending upon the system of weaning, milk removal through milking can be complete or partial. In complete milking entire milk is removed by milking process, while in partial milking, some proportion of milk is sucked by the calf and the remaining portion only is milked out. Depending upon the method adopted for, milking can be two types such as hand milking and machine milking. As the name indicates, hand milking (manual milking) is done with hands only, while machine milking is done using milking machine.

Hand Milking

This is done by squeezing the teat in between fingers of the hand so that pressure inside the udder increases widening the pressure difference between outside the udder. When pressure difference becomes sufficient to overcome the pressure exerted by sphincter muscles so as to keep the streak canal closed, milk flows out. Hand milking can be done in three ways based on the positioning of fingers and mode of pressure application such as Full hand milking, Stripping and Thumbing (knuckling).

In full hand milking top of the teat is locked between thumb and index finger and then pressure is exerted on the teat using other fingers so that milk ejects out. This is practiced when teat is sufficiently large and teat orifice is less tight. Stripping also involves locking the two fingers in similar way and then pulling the fingers downwards so that milk is squeezed out. Stripping is usually done when teats are small and tight and also at the beginning and end of milking by other methods, since stripping enables complete extraction of milk and milking of teat with narrow orifice. Full hand milking is considered as the most scientific method of milking since pressure is applied uniformly on the udder tissue so that it causes least injury to the udder tissue and minimum discomfort to the animal. However in situations where full hand milking is difficult due to small size of the teat or tight sphincter muscle, stripping is recommended.

Thumbing or knuckling is also widely practised by milkmen as it enables easier and faster milking though is not recommended for the damage produced to mammary tissues. In this method thumb is bent on to the teat and pressure is applied against remaining fingers on the other side of teat with downward pulling. Pointed pressure of knuckle region enables easier extraction of milk, but it causes varying degrees of internal damage to teat and its subsequent complications like teat obstruction and mastitis.

Machine Milking

Milking with help of milking machine is followed in dairy farms in order to reduce labour requirement when large number of high yielding dairy cows has to be milked. Depending upon the number of animals to be milked, milking machine can be smaller portable units with individual suction source for each milking unit or larger fixed units with centralised suction device. Principle of machine milking is intermittent application of negative and positive pressure

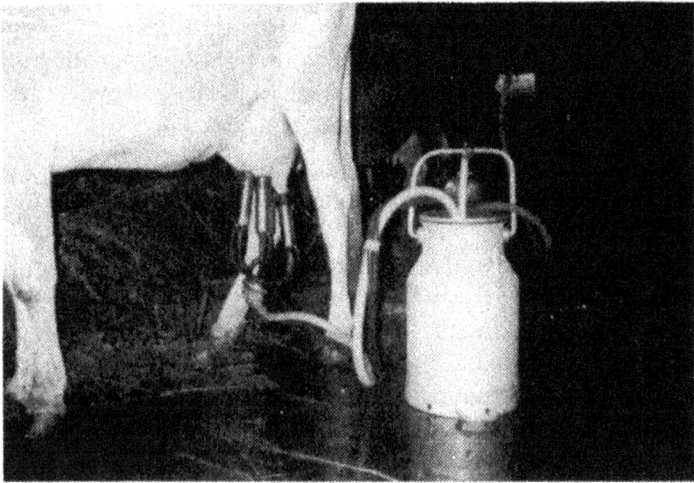
Fig. 6: Cow being milked using
milking machine

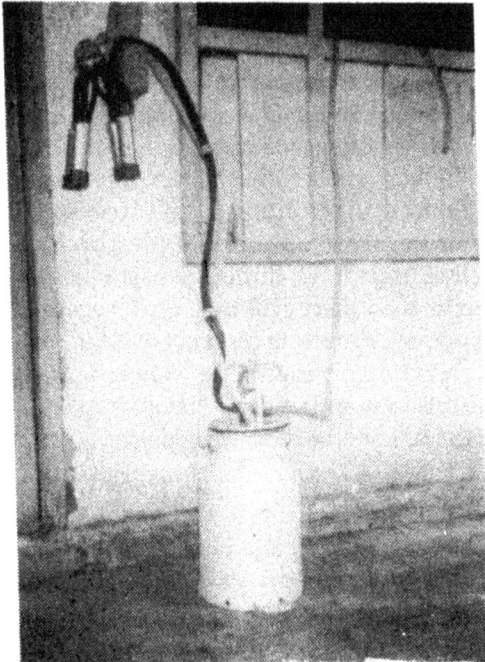
Fig. 7: Parts of an individual
milking machine unit

on the teat. Hence the process is more or less similar that of calf sucking milk from the udder, where in negative pressure is created by a suction pump and is applied on to the teats alternating with normal (positive) pressure at pre-fixed frequencies with the help of a pulsator and other parts of milking machine.

Parts of milking machine include suction pump, pulsator, teat cups, milk collecting can and connecting tubes. Suction pump forms the source of negative pressure, which can be centralised as seen in large dairy farms or individual units used in smaller milking units intended for fewer cows. Quantum of negative pressure can be regulated by adjustments on the suction pump or suction line. Pulsator is also called as the heart of milking machine since it has the vital role of alternating negative and normal pressure applied on to the teats through teat cups. Number of times of pressure alteration occurring during unit time can be adjusted by regulating frequency setting of the pulsator. Usually the frequency used is 50 - 60 and can vary between 40 -120 cycles per minute. Pulsator is usually connected to the suction source by a flexible rubber tube provided with valve for opening and closing.

Teat cups are four in number and are made of steel and provided with thin rubber liner. Free end of rubber liner is so arranged to suit teats of any size. Suction is usually applied into the gap between metallic portion and rubber liner of teat cups so that rubber liner expands and shrinks according to the frequency of pulsation. Alternation of negative and normal pressure generated at the pulsator reaches the teat cup through a pair of flexible rubber tubes connected to it. Also there will be a third tube, usually made of transparent plastic connecting centre of teat cups to the milk can or other milk collecting arrangements. Some amount of suction is allowed into this tube and milk can, in order to facilitate collection of milk into the can or other collecting places.

Milk can provided with suitable lid for air tight closure is used in smaller units of milking machine. Usually the pulsator will be fixed on this lid. Suction opened into the can from pulsator causes tight closure of the can and draws the entire milk entering the teat cups into this can. After milking and release of suction milk can be collected from the can and recording of individual animal's production can be done. In centralised automatic milking machine used in large dairies, there will be no milk can and milk from each milking unit goes straight away into the chilling plant. However there will be facility for recording the production of individual animal, taking samples, and for discarding milk of poor quality coming from diseased animals.

Advantage of Machine Milking

1. Considerable amount of labour can be saved and helps to minimise cost of production.
2. Enables quicker and hygienic milking, with minimum contamination
3. Since few animals can be milked simultaneously, saves time.
4. Minimises damage to udder tissue and reduces udder ailments
5. Provides better show to the milking process

Disadvantages Include

1. Requires high initial investment and maintenance cost
2. Complete milking is not possible, invariably necessitating stripping at beginning and end
3. Certain cows will not co operate with machine milking
4. Milk from individual quarters cannot be obtained or discarded separately
5. Improper cleaning of the machine deteriorates milk quality.

Healthy Milking Practices

Scientific milking practices helps to maintain udder health and better milk production with respect to quantity and quality of milk. Milking has to be carried out at regular timings with skilled persons preferably in milking parlours. As par as possible, change of milker and location has to be avoided. Before commencement of milking hindquarter and udder of the animal has to be washed to remove dung and dirt. The udder and surroundings has to moped dry with a clean towel to avoid dripping of wash water during milking. Animals can be fed with concentrate or green fodder in order to keep them quiet. However dusty feeds should not be offered at milking. Hind limbs and tail of the animal can be controlled with a rope

(8 knot) and proper precautions have to be taken in case of kicking animals.

Animal should not be frightened during milking. Wherever possible complete weaning has to be practised and intermittent suckling of calf has to be avoided. If required sterile lubricants can be smeared on the teats in order to minimise damage to tissues and easy millking. Milking has to be done as quick as possible once letting down takes place. Wherever possible full hand milking has to be adopted and thumbing should be avoided. Complete removal of milk has to be ensured and then udder has to be washed with water mixed with antiseptics and teat dipping has to be done if practised as a routine procedure.

Upon completion of milking milk has to be transferred quickly from the milking pail into the collecting vessel after recording the weight, preferably through suitable strainers. Milkers should follow clean habits and should avoid chewing, smoking and excessive talking at milking. Dust and Insects has to be controlled inside the milking parlour. After milking all utensils used for milking and the machine has to be thoroughly washed with clean water using suitable detergents in order to remove the residue of milk sticking on to them and to prevent microbial growth. Residue of washed water has to be drained out properly and the utensils have to be properly dried and kept in clean premises for usage at next milking.

Chapter 9
MILK AND ITS PROPERTIES

In the diet of every nation, milk is an indispensable food item and is considered as nature's perfect food for human beings as well as other animals. Mammals secretes milk for the nourishment of their young ones and milk of animals like cattle, buffalo, goat, sheep, camel, yak, llama, mithun, mare etc are being used as food for human beings. Of these animals cattle, buffalo and goat are the commonly reared dairy animals and the term 'Milk' in India often refers to milk of these animals. Dairy industry depends entirely on the ability of animals to produce milk for human consumption.

Milk may be defined as the whole, fresh, clean lacteal secretion obtained by the complete milking of one or more healthy milch animals, excluding that obtained within 15 days before or 5days after calving. Milk should be practically colostrum free and should contain the minimum prescribed percentages of milk fat and milk solids not fat (MSNF). Even though milk of different species contains almost same chemical constituents, proportion of the constituents varies. Hence properties and nutritive vlaue of milk vary widely between species and even between animals of same species to some extend.

Composition of Milk

Major constituents of milk are water, fat, protein, lactose, and mineral (ash). Minor milk constituents include phospholipids, sterols, vitamins, enzymes, pigments etc. All the constituents excluding water is usually denoted by the term total solids, which in turn is usually categorised into fat and solids not fat (SNF). Various chemical constituents of milk and their average proportion in cows milk is as follows:

Table 13

Organic Constituents	Percentage	Inorganic Constituents	Percentage
Lactose	4.9	Water	87
Lactalbumen	0.52	Calcium	0.12
Lactoglobulin	0.20	Phosphorus	0.10
Neutral fat	3.70	Sodium	0.05
Phospholipids	0.10	Potassium	0.15
Citric acid	0.20	Chlorine	0.11

PFA Standard for Milk

According to the Prevention of Food Adulteration Act (PFA) Rules, 1976, standards for different classes of milk throughout India vary according to the locality. In Kerala the following standards are prescribed.

Table 14

	Fat (%)	MSNF (%)
Cow milk	3.5	8.5
Buffalo milk	5	9
Goat milk	3.5	9

Factors Influencing Composition of Milk

Milk differs widely in composition according to different factors. All milk contain same kind of constituents but in varying amounts. Milk from individual cows show greater variation than mixed herd milk and the variation is always greater in small herds than in larger ones. Milk fat shows the greatest daily variation followed by protein, lactose and ash. Milk yield has got an inverse relationship with fat and protein content of milk. Thus high yielding animals will produce low fat milk and vice versa. Yield of milk increases gradually from the beginning and become maximal between 30-45 days and then decreases towards the end of lactation. Similarly lactose and chloride content are inversely related. Towards ‹ nd of lactation the lactose content decreases whereas chloridₑ content increases. This contributes to the salty taste of milk towards the end of lactation. Besides this composition of milk is affected by various factors such as:

Species of Animal

Each species of animal yield milk of characteristic composition. Proportion of major constituents in milk of different species is given below.

Table 15

Species	Water (%)	Fat (%)	Protein (%)	Lactose (%)	Ash (%)
Human	87.7	3.6	1.8	6.8	0.1
Cow	87.2	3.8	3.5	4.8	0.7
Buffalo	82.3	7.6	4.3	4.8	0.9
Goat	87.8	3.8	3.2	4.5	0.5

Breed

Breed is an important hereditary factor, which influence the composition of milk. High yielding breeds produce less fat and vice versa. Variations in composition of milk produced by Holstein and Jersey breeds as noted below:

Table 1ᵉ

Breed	Water	Total solids	Fat	Protein	Lactose	Ash
Holstein	88.07	11.93	3.45	3.15	4.65	0.68
Jersey	85.45	14.55	4.98	3.84	4.98	0.75

Individuality

Each cow yield milk of a composition that is characteristic of the individual and is different from milk produced by other cows under similar management situations.

Stage of Lactation

The milk yield and composition will vary based on the stage of lactation. Colostrum - first secretion after calving is entirely different from that of normal milk in its composition. Towards the end of lactation fat % and chloride content of milk increases and lactose content decreases.

Number of Milking

Three times milking of cows increases daily milk production by 10-25% compared to those milked twice daily and accordingly the composition also varies.

Age

Max.mum yield is obtained during second and third lactation and milk yield decreases during the subsequent lactations corresponding to the advancement of age. According to the yield composition especially fat percentage shows variations with age.

Seasonal Variations

The milk fat and quantity of milk are inversely proportional to the atmospheric temperature. That is milk production and fat percentage is more in both cold and rainy seasons. The same decrease in summer.

Feed

The quality and quantity of feed has a profound effect on the composition of milk given by the animal. Especially the feed affects fat percentage and character of the fat.

Interval of Milking

Longer interval is associated with more milk having a lower fat %.

Portion of Milking

Foremilk is low in fat content while strippings are highest

Excitement

Yield and composition of milk shows sudden fluctuations during excitement.

Disease and Abnormal Conditions

These tends to alter the copostion of milk especially when they result in a fall in milk yield.

Administration of Drugs and Hormones

Certain drugs causes temporary change in fat % and injection or feeding of certain hormones result in increase of both milk yield and fat%.

Major Milk Constituents .

Water

It exists in a continuous phase in which other milk constituents are either dissolved or suspended. Most of the water in milk is found in free form and only a very small portion is in the bound form (bound by milk protein, phospholipids etc.).

Fat

The bulk of the fat in milk exists in the form of small globules, called fat globules They have sizes ranging from 0.1 to 22 microns and is dispersed as oil in water type emulsion. The surface of each fat globule is coated with an adsorbed layer of material, called fat globular membrane. This membrane consists a phospholipid-protein complex that stabilises fat emulsion by keeping the globules separately. When milk is kept undisturbed, the fat globules tend to rise to the top of milk forming a cream layer. This is due to the lowest density of fat among milk constituents. Chemically milk fat is made up of tri glycerides(esters of fatty acids and glycerol). Most of the fatty acids of milk fat are saturated fatty acids and are relatively stable. Even though the unsaturated fatty acids are less in number they play an important role in the physico- chemical properties of milk fat.

Proteins

Like any other protein milk proteins are also composed of various essential and non-essential amino acids. In milk, protein exists as colloidal suspension. Mainly there are 3 types of milk proteins such as casein, α- lactalbumin and β-lacto globulin. Casein contributes more than 80 % of milk protein and lactalbumen contributes another 18 % and the remaining portion only is formed by lactoglobulin. It can be coagulated from milk by dilute acids, rennin and alcohol. Therefore it is known as coagulated milk protein. It is mainly associated with calcium salts present in milk. Other two milk proteins are found in whey (un-coagulated portion of milk).

Hence called as whey proteins. Proportions of these proteins are more in colostrum.

Lactose

It is the sugar seen only in milk and hence called as milk sugar. In milk lactose exists in true solution. Chemically lactose is composed of one molecule each of glucose and galactose. Milk is the only source of galactose in the food. Souring of milk is due to the production of lactic acid from lactose by lactose fermenting bacteria and it is important in the preparation of fermented milk products.

Mineral Matter or Ash

The mineral matter or salts of milk although present in small quantities, exert considerable influence on the physicochemical properties and nutritive value of milk. Major salts (present in appreciable quantities include) Potassium, Sodium, Magnesium, Calcium, Phosphorus, Citrate, Chloride, Sulphate, and Bicarbonate. Trace minerals include all other salts or minerals present in minute quantities. Part of the minerals occurs in true solution, while remaining portion exists in colloidal state.

Minor Milk Constituents

Phospholipids

In milk there are 3 types ot phospholipids such as lecithin, cephalin and sphingomyelin. They are found in fat globular membrane in association with protein. Phospholipids are excellent emulsifying agents and stabilise the milk fat emulsion.

Cholesterol

They are associated with fat globular membrane and non fat portion of milk and protein. Milk usually contains 0.1 g cholesterol per litre of milk.

Pigments

Milk contains various colouring pigments like Carotene, Xanthophil, Riboflavin, etc. Carotene is fat-soluble and is responsible for yellow colour of milk and other fat rich products. Riboflavin belongs B complex vitamin, which is a water-soluble greenish yellow pigment giving characteristic greenish yellow colour to whey.

Enzymes

Important enzymes normally present in milk are Lipase (fat splitting), Protease (protein splitting), Phosphatase (splitting phosphoric acid esters), Peroxidase and catalase (decomposes hydrogen peroxide), amylase (starch splitting) etc. They are proteins having specific action and are inactivated by heat.

Vitamins

Even though vitamins are present in very minute quantities in milk, they are vital for health and growth of living organisms. Important vitamins in milk are fat-soluble vitamin A, D, E and K and water-soluble vitamins of B complex group. Milk is normally deficient in vitamin C.

Physicochemical Properties of Milk

Being a complex solution of various organic and inorganic constituents, milk has got certain physicochemical properties. They are as follows:

The Physical State

In milk lactose and portion of mineral salts are found in true solution, proteins and reminder of minerals in colloidal suspension and fat as an emulsion. Water is the continuous phase in which the above constituents are either dissolved or suspended

Acidity and pH of Milk

The acidity of freshly drawn milk is called natural or apparent acidity and is caused by the presence of casein, acid phosphate, citrate etc in milk. This acidity varies depending upon species, breed, individuality, stage of lactation, physiological condition of udder etc. Higher the SNF content in milk, higher will be the natural acidity and vice versa. Natural acidity varies on an average from 0.13 to 0.14 per cent for cow milk and 0.14 to 0.15 per cent for buffalo milk. When milk is held at room temperature for some time its acidity increases as time goes on, which is due to the conversion of lactose into lactic acid by bacterial action. This acidity is known as 'developed' or 'real acidity'. There for titratable acidity of stored milk is equal to the sum of natural acidity and developed acidity and is expressed as 'percentage of lactic acid'.

The pH of freshly drawn milk varies from 6.4 - 6.6 for cow milk and 6.7- 6.8 for buffalo milk. Higher and lower pH values for fresh milk indicate udder infection and bacterial action respectively.

Specific Gravity

The mass of a substance per unit volume is known as density and the ratio of its density to density of water is known as specific gravity. As the specific gravity of a substance varies with temperature, it is necessary to specify the temperature when reporting density or specific gravity.

Since milk is heavier than water its density or specific gravity is more than that of water. Average specific gravity of milk at 15 °C ranges from 1.028 to 1.030 for cow milk and 1.030 to 1.032 for buffalo milk. The specific gravity is influenced by the composition of milk. Specific gravity of individual milk constituents varies and milk fat is the lightest component (0.93) while minerals are the heaviest (4.12). The specific gravity of milk is determined using lactometer.

Boiling Point of Milk

It is slightly higher than that of water and is around 100.17 °C or 212.3 °F

Freezing Point

Milk freezes at temperatures slightly lower than water due to the presence of soluble constituents such as lactose, soluble salts etc, which lower the freezing point. Average freezing point of cow milk is -0.547 °C and that of buffalo milk is -0.549 °C. Freezing point depression lower than this value indicates addition of water in milk.

Refractive Index

It is the degree of refraction (Path deviation) taking place when light passes from one medium to other. Refractive index of milk is slightly higher than that of water and value ranges from 1.3458 - 1.3478.

Viscosity

It is a measure of resistance to flow exhibited by fluids. Viscosity of milk ranges between 1.5 - 2 Cent poise.

Colour

The milk appears entirely opaque in large quantities while it is somewhat transparent in thin layers. Colour of milk varies from bluish white of buffalo milk to almost golden yellow of cow milk. The colour is a blend of individual colour produced by 1) Scattering of light - on colloidal casein particle and dispersed fat globule, which is responsible for the white colour of milk. 2) Carotene, which imparts a yellowish tinge.

Dairy animals differ in their capacity to transfer carotene from feed to milk fat depending upon the species, breed and individuality. Cows transfers more carotene into milk than buffaloes, leading to more yellowish colour of cow milk whereas buffalo milk is more whitish in colour. The intensity of yellow colour of cow milk depends on various factors such as breed, feed, size of fat globule fat % etc. Greater the intake of green fodder, deeper will be the yellowish colour. Larger the fat globule and higher the fat %, greater will be the intensity of yellow colour.

Flavour

Flavour is composed of smell (odour) and taste. The flavour of milk is a blend of the sweet taste of lactose and salty taste of minerals, both of which are damped down by proteins. The milk 'at also contributes to the characteristic rich flavour of milk. Changes in flavour of milk occur due to type of feed, season, stage of lactation, condition of udder, sanitation during milking, subsequent handling of milk and during storage. The sulphydril compounds significantly contributes to the cooked flavour of heated milk.

Food and Nutritive Value

Milk is nearly a complete food for human beings. It provides almost all essential nutrients such as body building proteins, bone forming minerals, health giving vitamins and energy giving lactose and milk fat. It contains all these nutrients in an easily digestible and assimilable form. Therefore milk is an important food for all categories of persons such as pregnant and lactating mothers growing children, aged persons, patients etc.

Milk protein contains all the essential amino acids in fairly large quantities. Milk is an excellent source of calcium and phosphorus and these are essential for bone and teeth formation.

Milk is rather low in Iron, Copper and Iodine. Vitamins are essential nutrients, which support normal growth of human body. Milk is a good source of all fat soluble vitamins. Milk also contain B complex vitamins and milk is deficient in vitamin C. Milk fat serve as a rich source of energy and place a significant role in the nutritive value, flavour and physicochemical properties of milk and milk products. Milk fat contains all essential fatty acids. It gives rich pleasing flavour, which is not duplicated by any other type of fat. Principal function of milk lactose is to supply energy. Also it helps to establish a mild acidic reaction in intestine, which checks the growth of proteolytic bacteria and facilitate assimilation. Energy value of milk varies depending upon its composition. On an average cow milk furnishes 75 Kilo calories per 100 gram and buffalo milk 100 Kilo calories per 100 gram. Energy value of individual milk constituents is as follows:

Table 17

Milk fat	9.3 K. Cal/g.
Milk protein	4.1 K. Cal/g.
Milk sugar	4.1 K. Cal/g.

Adulterants and Preservative in Milk

Adulterants are those substances added to milk for the purpose of cheating through modifying the quantity or quality of milk. The common adulterants of milk are water, sugar, starch, skim milk powder, colouring matter etc. Of these water is the chief adulterant of milk. Addition of water to milk may be suspected if the specific gravity goes below 1.027, the total solids of milk decreases below 11 % and the freezing point come near to 0. Of these specific gravity and total solids can vary depending upon many natural or artificial reasons. However freezing point is remarkably a constant and cannot be altered by any other factors other than addition of water. Hence freezing point is considered as the actual index for detecting adulteration of milk with water.

Sugar is commonly added to milk in order to increase the specific gravity of milk and thus to increase the lactometer reading, which is an essential factor for determining the SNF content of milk during pricing. The added sugar can be detected using Seliwanoff's test. When milk is mixed and boiled for 5 minutes with Seliwanoff's reagent (1 ml of conc. HCL and 100 mg Resorcinol powder), a red colour is developed, if sugar is present.

Addition of starch into milk increases the thickness of milk. For detecting starch adulteration, commonly employed test is iodine test. Here a small quantity of milk is boiled and cooled. Then a drop of iodine solution is added into it. A blue colour indicates presence of starch.

Preservatives are those substances added to milk in order to increase the keeping quality of milk. Addition of preservatives into milk is not legally permitted. Preservatives are normally added to milk samples preserved at room temperature for laboratory analysis. Commonly added preservatives are hydrogen peroxide, mercuric chloride, Boric acid, bleaching powder etc. Detection of preservatives can be carried out by specific tests for each of them.

Colostrum

It is the mammary secretion obtained during initial period of lactation (usually 3-4 days). Colostrum is reddish yellow in colour (sometime referred as "liquid gold"), usually having an abnormal odour, bitter taste and is very slimy, viscous, and acidic. Colostrum is entirely different from that of milk with regard to its composition and physicochemical properties. Because of its high total solids, colostrum has a high specific gravity (1.07) than normal milk. Usual composition is as follows:

Table 18

Water	71.3 %,
Total solids	28.7 %
Fat	3.8%
Protein - 20.6 % (Casein - 4.8 %, Albumen and globulin - 15.8 %)	
Sugar	2.2 %
Ash	1.7 %,

Microscopically colostrums shows a large number of colostral cells, which might be due to either sloughing of epithelial cells of udder or engorgement of leucocytes by absorption of fat globules. Fat globules in colostrums are large and irregularly shaped while those of milk are round.

Importance

Colostrum contains more globulin and albumen than normal milk and it is important for developing immunity against several diseases. Colostral antibodies are absorbed directly from the intestine without much chemical alteration, immediately after birth. However permeability of intestinal mucosa to colostral antibodies decreases rapidly as time goes on. Hence colostrum feeding has to be done to new born calves preferably within half to one hour.

Colostrum contains much more vitamins especially Vitamin A (in the form of carotene), which also contributes to high disease resistance of calves. High mineral content in colostrums is helpful in the formation of bone and teeth favouring better health and growth rate. Colostrum is also a good laxative stimulating the functioning of intestinal tract and facilitating passing out of meconium (first faecal matter - formed in intestine during its growth inside the uterus). Due to high content of minerals colostrum has a tendency to coagulate easily upon heating. This facilitates differentiation of colostrums from normal milk, besides differences in colour and consistency.

Usually colostrum is not used for human consumption and surplus quantity after feeding calf goes wasted. However it is of very high nutritive value due to its rich chemical composition and can be used for human consumption by converting into suitable products. Surplus colostrum also can be used for feeding other calves or even other animals either fresh or after preservation as fermented colostrum.

Milk of Other Species

Besides cow, buffalo and goat are the most commonly reared dairy species. Among these buffaloes are the major milk producers in India, while goats contributes only around 2 % of total milk production. Physicochemical properties of buffalo milk and goat milk are similar to cow milk in most respects and variation in chemical composition has already been described. Striking differences of buffalo milk and goat milk from cow milk includes

Buffalo Milk

Colour of buffalo milk is pure white due to the absence of carotene pigment unlike in the case of cow milk. Also it is thicker in consistency due to high content of milk solids, viz., fat, proteins, lactose and minerals. Buffalo milk normally has a higher pH, acidity, buffer value, density, viscosity and fat globule size than cow milk or goat milk. Compared to cow milk, casein content is more (3 per cent) and there exists distinct differences in physicochemical make up of casein from buffalo milk such as size, proportion, and solubility of casein micelles. Similarly Calcium and Phosphorus content is also more in buffalo milk with a high calcium: Phosphorus ratio. Besides higher proportion in milk, buffalo milk fat is different from cow milk with respect to the composition of fatty acids. Due to its high content of fat and higher yield, buffalo milk is preferred for ghee making. However ghee from buffalo milk is more whitish in colour and harder than that from cow milk.

Goat Milk

Consistency and composition of goat milk is more or less same as in cow milk, while the colour is pure white as in the case of buffalo milk. However goat milk usually have a peculiar 'Goatish odour" absorbed from its premises of production which forms a reason for dislike by some people. Fat in goat milk is dispersed as very small globules when compared to milk of other species. This contributes to better digestibility and hence goat milk is best for children and sick people. Due to smaller sized fat globules goat milk is used for production of soft cheese and other products.

Chapter 10
MICROBIOLOGICAL QUALITY OF MILK

Milk being highly nutritious, forms a good medium for bacterial growth and even with all precautions milk, immediately after drawing from the udder, contains large numbers of bacteria. Also bacterial count of milk rises very rapidly after milking depending upon the storage conditions. Low microbial count is very important in deciding the keeping quality of milk and to avoid deleterious effects caused by pathogenic organisms upon its consumption.

Microbiology of Milk

Nearly all changes taking place in the flavour and appearance of milk, after it is drawn from udder, are result of activities of micro organisms. Of these the most important one are bacteria, molds, yeasts and viruses and among this bacteria predominates. According to the changes produced in milk, they may be classified into desirable micro organisms (Those producing desirable changes in milk), undesirable micro organisms (those spoiling milk) and disease producing microorganisms or pathogens. Important microbial organisms seen in milk are:

Bacteria

Bacteria are unicellular organisms occurring principally in the form of spherical, cylindrical or spiral cells. In milk spherical and cylindrical forms are predominant. Most bacteria may be of 1-2 microns in size. Although individual bacterial cells are invisible to the naked eye, bacterial colonies (consists large number of individual cells) are visible. Under favourable conditions, bacteria multiply very rapidly and may double in their number in each 15 minutes or less. Some bacteria form "spores" under unfavourable conditions, which are tough resistant bodies within the bacterial cells. Thus spore-forming bacteria are able to overcome pasteurisation and even sterilisation temperatures. When spores are placed in an environment favourable for growth, they form new vegetative cells and starts multiplication again.

Bacteria normally present in milk are called natural flora of milk and includes species of Streptococcus, Lactococcus, Lactobacillus, Pseudomonas, Bacillus, etc.

Mold

They are multi-cellular micro organisms differing in most respects from bacteria. Although individual cells are not visible to the naked eye, at maturity they may be observed readily as mycelium. Even though molds also form spores for multiplication, most spores of molds present in milk are destroyed by pasteurisation temperature.

Yeast

They are also unicellular organisms but some what larger in size than bacteria. Spores of yeasts in milk are also readily destroyed during pasteurisation

Viruses

They are ultra microscopic forms of life. In milk only those viruses that are parasitic on lactic acid bacteria known as starter bacteriophages are of special importance, since lactic baceriophages are not destroyed by normal pasteurisation of milk. However, higher temperatures can destroy them easily.

Growth of Micro organisms

In microbiology, growth refers to increase in number. Milk drawn from a healthy cow already contains some bacteria. Their number multiplies during production and handling, depending on the cleanliness of these operations. Subsequently their numbers may grow further depending upon the storage conditions. The changes taking place in the physico chemical properties of milk are the result of activities of the individual microbial cells during their period of growth or of substances produced during such activity.

Factors influencing bacterial growth: Major factors are

Food Supply
Milk furnish all the nutrient requirement of microorganisms.

Moisture
Milk contains adequate moisture for their growth

Air
Milk supplies oxygen for the growth of aerobic type of bacteria

Temperature
Each species of micro organisms have its optimum temperature of growth.

Others
Other factors affecting growth are acidity, pH, preservative, light, concentration etc

According to the optimum temperature for growth, bacteria can be classified into:

Psychrotropic
They can grow at refrigeration temperatures (5-7 °C)

Mesophilic
Their optimum growth temperature ranges between 20 - 40 °C

Thermophilic (Heat loving)
They can grow at temperatures above 50 °C

Destruction of Micro Organisms

Micro organisms can be destroyed by heat, ionising radiation, high frequency sound waves, electricity, pressure, chemicals etc.

Results of Microbial Growth

During growth of micro organisms inside milk, they will utilise various milk constituents and produces new substances being by products or end products of their activity and thus changing original quality of milk. These changes can be beneficial sometime, while causes spoilage of milk otherwise depending upon the nature of change and products produced. Major changes produced by microbial growth in milk are the following:

Souring

This is a process of converting lactose in milk to lactic acid and other volatile acids by lactic acid bacteria.

Gas Production

This is caused mainly by coliform bacteria which are commonly found in soil, manure, feed etc. Presence of coliform in milk indicates contamination from the above sources.

Flavour Production

Both desirable and undesirable flavours in milk are produced by micro organisms. Desirable flavour is produced mainly from citrate present in milk. Undesirable flavours are produced by spoilage microorganisms.

Proteolysis

Protein in milk is decomposed by micro organisms to their simpler components and desirable and undesirable changes are produced.

Lipolysis

It is the decomposition of fat present in milk by micro organisms and produce mainly transient flavour.

Major benefit of microbial growth is lactic fermentation leading to production of various products. Products of microbial growth are enzymes, decomposition products of fat, protein and lactose, pigments, toxins etc. Similarly major defects produced by microbial growth include Gas production, abnormal flavour production (bitter, rancid, oxidised etc.), ropiness, sweet curdling, abnormal colour etc.

Clean Milk Production

During milking and handling utmost care should be taken to ensure quality especially microbial quality of milk. Even at the time of milking there will be lot of bacteria and other organisms inside the milk and microbial count of milk goes on increasing due to rapid multiplication of organisms already present as well due to introduction of more and more organisms via contamination. Upon multiplication these micro organisms goes on degrading milk constituents and deteriorate quality. Hence initial microbiological quality is very crucial in deciding the holding time available before

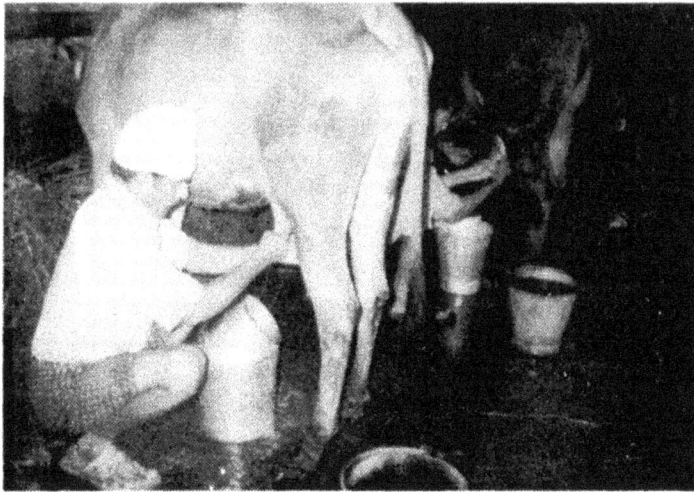

Fig. 8: Cow being hand milked into partly covered milking pail

processing and thus urgency of distribution and processing. Sources for bacterial contamination of freshly collected milk includes:

Animal Body

Cow's body harbours plenty of bacteria and other microbes which can gain access into the milk many ways. Contamination of milk from animal body can be from interior of udder itself, from those organisms residing inside the udder either as normal or pathological inhabitants. Bacterial count of milk in the udder can be high in case of sub-clinical infection or weakening of sphincter muscles guarding streak canal. Contamination can also occur while milking from the external aspect of udder or due to spillage of urine or dung, falling of hairs and dripping of water into the milk and so on.

Surroundings

Unhygienic surroundings can contribute to high bacterial count of milk via dropping of particles in a dusty atmosphere, falling or touching of insects like flies in to the milking vessels either before, during or after milking.

Milker

Hygienic practices of milker is also very important in determining bacterial quality of milk. Hands, nails, clothes, diseases and certain habits of milker such as smoking during milking, talking etc. enhance bacterial contamination of milk.

Utensils

Milking, handling of milk and processing requires various types of vessels and other utensils and all of this can be potent contributors of bacteria in to the milk unless they are thoroughly cleaned and sterilised.

Precautionary measures for minimising bacterial contamination and thus to ensure clean milk production are summarised in the following table:

Table 19

Sl. No	Source of Contamination	Precautionary measures
1.	Interior of udder	Thoroughly wash the udder before milking and mop dry. Discard fist few strippings of milk. Practice teat dipping with antiseptics after milking. Frequently screen for sub-clinical mastitis and treat the cases Treat systemic diseases if any
2.	Exterior of udder	Wash the hind quarters of the animal prior to milking. Wash the udder with antiseptics and water before milking. Dry the udder using a clean towel. Control the animal properly and tie the tail
3.	Surroundings	Avoid milking at damp places and dusty atmosphere. Avoid feeding of mashes during or just before milking. Use partly covered milking pails. Control insects
4.	Milker	Wash the hands thoroughly and cut nails. Avoid personnel with respiratory diseases from milking. Insist clean clothes and preferably face mask. Avoid habits like smoking and chewing during milking Insist scientific milking methods and complete milking
5.	Utensils	Store the utensils in clean and dry places. Thoroughly clean and sterilise using suitable methods. Avoid chances of post sterilisation contamination

Even with all these precautions we cannot eliminate bacteria from milk. Hence processing should be initiated as early as possible after milking in order to avoid quality deterioration from microbial action.

Bacteriological Standards of Raw Milk

In developed countries grading of milk is done based on bacteriological quality so that its keeping quality and safety for human consumption are more or less assured. However in our country such system for grading of milk quality is still in its infancy. As the beginning step in this direction, ISI I as prescribed the following bacteriological standards as a guide for grading raw milk.

Table 20

Sl.No.	Bacterial Number (expressed as SPC)	Grade
1.	Not exceeding 2 lakhs	Very good
2.	2-10 lakhs	Good
3.	10-50 lakhs	Fair
4.	Over 50 lakhs	Poor

Cleaning and Sanitation of Utensils

Under ordinary farm conditions, utensils are the greatest single source of bacteria and often contribute large numbers of organisms to an otherwise high quality milk. Milk is brought into contact with a great variety of utensils from the time it leaves the cow until it is placed before the consumer. Hence clean, sanitised and dry utensils are absolute necessities in the production of milk with a low bacterial content and high keeping quality.

The utensils must be rinsed, washed, and sanitised as soon as possible after they have been used. Metal utensils such as pails, cans, strainer, etc should be rinsed with cold water or lukewarm water after each milking. This removes much of the milk and after this, they should be washed and scrubbed with a brush and using plenty of clean water preferably warm to which some detergent or washing powder has been added. This is necessary to get the utensils rid of the film of fat. Then they should be rinsed with plenty of warm water or hot water before being sanitized.

Sanitising is done by means of hot water, steam, or chemicals such as chlorine solutions of one kind or another. The hot water or steam is preferred, however if these are not available one may resort to the use of chemicals like hypochlorite or chloramine solutions. These are quite effective if they have the proper amount of available chlorine during usage and when utensils are cleaned thoroughly. Strainer clothes if used should be washed, boiled, and dried after each milking and preferably a new filter disc should be used at each milking.

Chapter 11
MILK COLLECTION AND HANDLING

In India dairy industry is not organised as in developed countries and organised dairy farms are very few in number. Major proportion of milk is produced in household dairy units in villages having 2-3 numbers of cattle or buffaloes. Through the establishment of dairy co-operatives, organising of small scale dairy farmers has become possible. Dairy cooperatives collect milk produced by the farmers through their collection centres (societies), transport to regional processing plants (dairy plants) and distribute to consumers especially in urban areas through organised retail outlets. The entire process involves varying levels of transportation and storage before delivering processed milk to demand centres.

Procurement of Milk

Most often in all countries production of milk is confined to rural areas, while its demand is mostly from urban centres. Milk produced in villages is collected through co operative societies or their collection booth set up in centres of better milk production. In some cases collection is carried out by contractors and supply to dairies, or the producers in the vicinity supplies the milk produced themselves to the dairy plants. Contractors involved in milk collection act as middlemen and gives less price to the producer so as to make their profit.

In Kerala most of the milk collecting societies are functioning under respective regional milk unions and such societies are

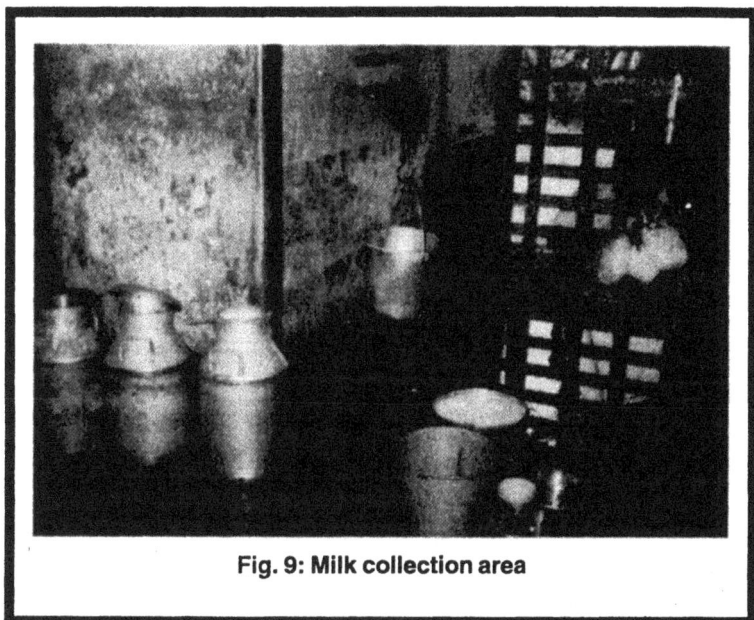

Fig. 9: Milk collection area

designated as "Anand pattern co operative societies" or APCOS. These societies have got similar pattern of functioning and they provide various benefits to its members besides milk marketing facility. Usually the supplying members will be enrolled as members of the society and some among them are also nominated to its board of management. However there are some private societies also collecting and distributing milk at different localities usually called as traditional societies.

In co-operative societies, milk collection is usually carried out twice in a day coinciding with prevailing milking times of the locality such as early morning and afternoon. The individual producer has to supply the milk at these centres as early as possible after milking. At the time of collection samples will be taken for testing fat and pricing is usually done based on the fat content.

Pricing of Milk

Pricing of milk is rather complicated due to the possibility of adulteration and is of concern to the producers, distributors and processors. All these categories of people have different levels of costs involved and like to have a margin of profit after covering the costs. Since high level of profit taken by one category adversely affects others, there is need for an integrated and sound pricing policy, which is acceptable to all concerned. An effective pricing policy has the following aims:

1. Safeguards the interests of producers, processors, distributors and consumers
2. Guarantees better price and market for milk throughout the year
3. Forms an incentive to produce more milk by the producers
4. Enables consumers to get wholesome milk at reasonable rates
5. Leave an attractive and reasonable margin of profit to the processors

In order to encourage production of better quality cow milk, National Dairy Development Board introduced the policy of two axis pricing system based on the relative values of fat and SNF in milk. Such a system ensures payment of milk based on its compositional quality and discourages adulteration of milk with water and also ensures equivalent pricing for cow and buffalo milk. Based on the past experiences on the proportions of fat and SNF in milk, a chart is prepared for ready payment of milk by evaluating fat and taking price of SNF as 2/3 rd that of price of fat.

For *e.g.*, Suppose price of 1 Kg fat is Rs 120, from two axis price chart 10 Kg of buffalo milk containing 6 % fat and 9 % SNF will get Rs 72 for its fat content and Rs 72 for its SNF content so that total price of that milk come Rs 144.00. While 10 Kg cow milk having 4.5 % fat and 8.6 % SNF will get Rs 54 for its fat content and Rs 68.8 for its SNF making a total price of Rs 122.80. Price rates of the chart vary according to the region and time. As the commodity prices are increasing in the market, changes have to be made in the price rates so that necessary hike occurs for milk price also.

Chilling Plants

Milk being highly perishable commodity, milk collected has to be processed at the earliest in order to minimise quality deterioration. If time required for reaching the dairy is less direct shipment of raw milk can be done. However if the distance from collection centres to the processing plants are more, or more time is required for other reasons, milk has to be cooled before transporting to processing plants. For this, chilling plants are established at convenient places, wherein milk from the nearby locality are cooled and transported to dairy plants. Usually chilling plants are owned by producers' co-operative organisations of the locality or the milk distributors and accordingly their functioning may vary.

Milk brought in by larger producers and milk societies are received after necessary steps, weighed, cooled and producer's cans are returned after washing. Milk is then cooled and stored at low temperature until it is despatched to processing dairies. Transportation is usually carried out in road or rail tankers or in cans depending upon the quantity and distance to be transported. Collecting milk at chilling plants has certain advantages over direct collection at dairies such as:

1. Enables transport of better quality milk to dairies
2. Only few cans are required for the producer or societies
3. Less chance of losing cans and less damage to cans
4. Payment to producers are direct and fast
5. Producer can observe weighing and testing and avoids dispute
6. Since cooling is done collectively, reduces expenditure for this

Chilling plants are located in places where there is adequate milk production, availability of sufficient water, electricity, transportation facilities such as road and proximity to railway and waste disposal facilities. Equipments required include milk weighing tank with weighing scale, drop tank (dump tank) with cover, storage tank, can washer, milk pump, surface or plate cooler, refrigeration unit, cold room and milk testing unit.

Milk received at the chilling plant is cooled below 20 °C and ISI has prescribed a temperature of 10 °C and below. Purpose of this is that milk when drawn from the udder, invariably contains some micro -organisms and further there will be increase in the number due to contamination during subsequent handling. These micro-organisms further multiply and grow faster especially when the temperature is between 20 - 40 °C and in turn causes deterioration of milk quality. Bacterial multiplication is inhibited by low temperature and hence the milk is cooled to around 4-5 °C so as to minimise deterioration.

Methods of cooling adopted in chilling plants is by using different types of coolers such as immersion coolers, bulk milk coolers, surface coolers, plate milk coolers and so on. In immersion cooler, a small portable refrigeration system is immersed in milk and is suitable for cooling small quantity of milk. Bulk milk coolers involve an insulated milk storage tank provided with cooling device so that large quantity of milk can be cooled at a time. In surface coolers milk is poured over a cooling tube through which there will be continuous flow of cold water or other cooling medium and the chilled milk is collected in a tank. Plate type coolers have plate type heat exchangers as in the case of HTST pasteuriser and are suitable for chilling of large quantities only.

Transportation

Different methods of transportation are adopted depending upon the quantity and distance of milk to be transported. In rural areas for transporting small quantities methods like head load, shoulder sling, carriage by pet animals, bullock cart and tonga are commonly used. While for larger quantities and long distances milk is transported by motor truck, road and rail tankers. Within a radius of 50 KMs milk can be transported in ordinary milk cans carried on lorries or trucks. If the distance is more than 50 KMs milk has to be chilled and carried in milk tankers or thermo can lorries. Use of milk can is now a days limited to transport from milk producers to collection centres.

Milk transported beyond a distance of 300 KMs has to be pasteurised and sent by thermo-can lorries. Long distance transportation requires tankers like refrigerated tanker lorries for making transportation more economic and reducing deterioration of quality. Larger tankers also minimise contamination and enables better refrigeration so that better bacterial quality is assured.

For very long distances and larger quantity rail tankers can be used, which is cheaper than road tankers over large distance and quantity. For usual transportation (around 1000 KMs) rail tankers cause more expenditure and is inconvenient since there will be extra expenditures for loading and unloading, few tanker lorries are usually needed at loading and unloading, there will be delay due to booking and other formalities and so on. Hence lorry tankers are the best for transporting milk for long distances even though initial investment is high.

Receiving Milk at Dairy Plant

Upon arrival of milk at chilling plant or processing dairies, milk is subjected to certain preliminary examination in order to assess its general quality and decide whether to accept or reject. At point of reception milk should be clean, sweet, with pleasant flavour, free from off flavours and reasonably free from extraneous material. Sanitary quality of milk on receiving platform depends on its production situation at the farm and situations of handling and transportation. Milk may be arriving in cans or tankers and before emptying, the milk is inspected for gross changes in organoleptic quality and is done to find whether a particular lot of milk is fit for processing or not.

Milk cans are unloaded from the vehicle and are taken to emptying points, where the lids are removed and milk is inspected. If there is no gross abnormality of quality, milk is poured into a weighing tank and the weight is recorded. Simultaneously a sample of milk will be collected for detailed testing of quality. Emptied can and its lid are then taken to can washer. From the weighing tank milk is then transferred to a dump tank and from which pumping of milk is done in to a raw milk storage tank kept at higher level to permit gravity flow to pasteuriser.

Milk coming in tankers is also thoroughly inspected for quality. For unloading outlets of the tanker is connected to sanitary pipes and milk is then pumped into the storage tank. The tanker is then subjected to through washing and sanitation. Milk coming from chilling plants might be graded already, weighed, sampled and cooled. However milk is usually weighed and sampled again at central dairy in order to rule out any variation in the quantity and quality. In order to minimise deterioration of quality due to delay in processing, milk reception should be completed within 3 to 4 hours.

Chapter 12
QUALITY EVALUATION

Testing of quality is usually done based on a set of tests called platform tests. The platform test refers to all those tests, which are performed to check the quality of incoming milk on the receiving platform so as to make a quick decision regarding its acceptance or rejection. They are performed on each can or tanker of milk with the object of detecting milk of inferior or doubtful quality so as to prevent it being mixed with high-grade milk. The platform test includes tests for organoleptic quality, (Otherwise known as Rapid platform tests), sedimentation and acidity, lactometer reading, COB (Clot on boiling) test, Alcohol test, Alizarin-alcohol test etc. Of these organoleptic tests are applied to each can of milk and other tests might be used to substantiate the initial findings.

Organoleptic Tests

This include testing smell or odour, taste, appearance and temperature. Odour of milk is the most simple and valuable test to decide fitness of milk for processing. Lid of each can is removed, inverted and raised to the nose to receive the smell. The smell will be representative of the milk in the can. Then the milk is vigorously shaken using a plunger and smell is tested again. Sourness due to bacterial contamination can be identified by the smell and can be further confirmed, if required, by the taste as well. When there is excess of lactic acid and other volatile compounds formed out of lactose fermentation causes sourness to the smell. Excess acidity thus formed makes milk unfit for further processing since there will be lowering of coagulation temperature of casein.

Appearance

Appearance of milk should be inspected for any floating extraneous matter, colour change and partial curdling which are unusual in normal milk. Temperature of the milk coming from chilling plants should be checked. Temperature of more than 5°C indicates bacterial action and reflects quality.

Sedimentation

Test for sedimentation is a simple and rapid test to detect the extend of extraneous matter in the milk and presence of appreciable sediment excluding gross particles like hair, flies, pieces of hay or straw indicates careless or unsanitary practices at the farm. For this purpose a sediment tester is used.

Acidity

Titratable acidity of milk is used to ascertain whether the milk is fit for receiving heat treatment. Natural or apparent acidity does not make the milk sour, but developed acidity due to excess lactic acid, adversely affects the quality of milk and alters its behaviour upon heat treatment.

Lactometer Reading

Lactometer reading is another test to find out adulteration with water. However partial skimming and addition of thickening agents cannot be detected by lactometer. Hence estimation of fat and total solids will be required to confirm adulteration with water.

Clot on Boiling (COB) Test

This test is used to determine the heat stability of milk. If acidity of milk exceeds 0.17 %, that leads to appearance of clots on boiling.

Alcohol Test

It is an indication of the mineral balance of milk. It aids in detecting abnormal milk such as colostrum, milk from animals at late lactation or suffering from mastitis. Forth mentioned milk form clots by reacting with alcohol.

Alizarin-Alcohol Test

This is similar to the above tests, but it helps to indicate the approximate percentage of acidity.

Sampling

Collection of a representative sample for carrying out detailed evaluation of chemical and bacteriological quality is a very important step at milk reception. Material required for samlping includes a stirrer, sampling dipper and sample bottles. All these items should be clean, dry and sterile in order to get right picture of the milk based on the sample taken. For sampling the milk has to be thoroughly mixed using stirrer, or taking sample from the weighing tank so that milk will be mixed uniformly while pouring from the can. For larger tankers stirring can be done using a plunger operated manually or mechanically for sufficient time so as to ensure through mixing.

Usually about 50 ml of milk is collected as the sample and is kept tightly closed in sampling bottles until processing. Samples has to be properly labelled in order to avoid mixing of samples and resultant variations in quality assessed. Samples can be individual for each can or compartment of tanker or composite for the entire milk from same source. Samples for bacteriological examination has to be collected aseptically in sterile containers. Soon after collection samples are cooled by packing in ice and despatched to laboratory for testing. Samples from doubtful lots are tested in quality control laboratories for deciding the final acceptance or rejection. .

Laboratory Tests for Milk

All the dairy plants or collection centres should have a well equipped laboratory for routine determination of quality of raw milk as well as processed milk. Now a days electronic testing devices are available for testing certain routine qualities and can be employed wherever feasible. Every sample of milk is tested for fat and SNF and sample wise records are maintained for effecting payments. Periodic recordings regarding quality of milk taken in and processed milk sent out will help periodic evaluation of production and processing methods and to make necessary changes for improvement of quality of processed milk supplied and to ensure safety of the consumer.

Commonly done laboratory tests include testing of fat, SNF, detection of adulterants, and some bacteriological tests.

Testing of fat usually done using Gerber's method. In this method milk is mixed with Gerber's sulphuric acid in a Gerber's Butyrometer. All the contents other than fat are dissolved in the acid so that fat is separated. This separation process is also assisted by the exothermic reaction of the contents with acid. Amyl alcohol is also added into the mixture in order to avoid charring of fat. The mixture is then centrifuged so that a clear column of fat is formed inside the stem of butyrometer and length of the column can be read directly from the graduations on the butyrometer stem. Now a days in most of the dairy plants there is an electronic milk testing device called as "Milko-tester". It automatically give the fat percentage of each sample placed in it. SNF can be determined by the use of different formulae. For this lactometer reading and fat % of each sample has to be predetermined.

Detection of Adulterants

Common adulterants of milk are water, starch, sugar etc. Detection of water adulteration can be done determining freezing point. Freezing point is determined using an instrument called "cryoscope". Freezing of fresh milk is remarkably constant and adulteration with water results in a lowering of freezing point. Starch adulteration can be detected using Iodine test. In this test milk after boiling and subsequent cooling is mixed with iodine solution, so that development of a blue colour indicates the presence of starch as an adulterant. Presence of sugar can be detected using Seliwanoff's test. Here milk is mixed with Seliwanoff's reagent (mixture of conc. Hydrochloric acid and resorcinol) and boiled. Red colour indicates presence of sugar.

Bacteriological Quality

Bacteriological quality is tested using routine test such as:

1. Dye reduction test
2. Direct microscopic count
3. Standard plate count and
4. Examination of coliform organisms.

All these tests help to grade the milk into different grades so as to assess the quality of milk.

Dye Reduction Test

Dye reduction test involves testing the time required for reducing dyes such as methylene blue or resazurine. Colour of these dyes are altered by change in oxidation reduction potential of milk. Hence rate at which discharge of colour takes place is an indication of metabolic rate and thus bacterial activity of milk. Rate of colour change varies depending upon the type organisms present and their activity at a particular temperature. Greater the number of bacteria, shorter will be the time required for dye reduction and thus rate of dye reduction indicates quality of milk.

Methylene blue will give blue colour to milk and upon reduction the colour will disappear. If the disappearance of blue colour occurs within 30 minutes, such milk cannot be accepted. Based on this test milk can be graded as:

Table 21

M.B.R. Time	Grade
5 hours and above	Very good
Between 3 and 5 hours	Good
Between 1 and 3 hours	Fair
Below 1 hour	poor

In resazurin reduction test instead of methylene blue resazurin is being used, which is a more sensitive dye, hence requires only lesser time. Usually for resazurin reduction, tubes are incubated for only 10 minutes and the colour is compared with a resazurin disc in a comparator. Reading of 4 or more is considered satisfactory.

Direct Microscopic Count

Stained and dried film of milk prepared out of a measured volume is examined under a microscope and number of bacteria present in unit area is counted so as to estimate total bacterial count of milk. Usually 0.01 ml of milk is spread over an area of 1 square centimetre on a clean glass slide. The smear is then dried and stained suitably and average number of bacteria per microscopic field is counted under a microscope. Thus extend of bacterial contamination can be assessed and the milk sample can be classified into different grades. ISI standards for grading milk based on bacteriological quality assessed by direct microscopic count is as follows:

Table 22

Bacterial count per millilitre	Grade
Less than 500,000	Good
Between 500,000 to 4,000,000	Fair
Between 4,000,000 to 20,000,000	Poor
Over 20,000,000	Very poor

Besides assessment of quality, this test also enables tracing of probable source of contamination based on appearance of organisms. However this test gives accurate results only for high-count samples and is not suitable to test low count milk samples.

Standard Plate Count

This method is suitable for enumerating small number of bacteria, hence suitable for low count samples. Hence usually used for pasteurised milk or good quality raw milk. Here a measured volume of milk is inoculated into a agar gel after sufficient dilution. The plate is then incubated and number of colonies are counted for getting the count of bacteria and the actual count in the milk sample is assessed. As per ISI specification plate count of pasteurised milk should not exceed 50,000 per ml and ISI specification for raw milk is given below.

Table 23

Standard plate count	Grades
Below 200,000	Very good
Between 200,000 to 1,000,000	Good
Between 1,000,000 to 5,000,000	Fair
Over 5,000,000	Poor

Coliform Test

Coliform organisms are usually seen in raw milk as contamination from animal body and surroundings. For high grade milk, coliform organisms should not be present in 0.01 ml of milk. Coliform organisms are destroyed by pasteurisation. Hence they should not be present in 0.1 ml pasteurised milk and its presence indicates post pasteurisation contamination.

Chapter 13
PROCESSING OF MILK

Milk is a complete food as it contains various nutrients supporting life in more or less correct proportion and easily utilisable form. For the same reason milk is highly perishable commodity as well, since there will be rapid setting up and multiplication of various microorganisms, especially bacteria. Bacteria gains entry into the milk to some extent from the udder itself and thence even with all precautions there will be large number of bacteria in the milk. During and after milking there will occur entry of bacteria in to the milk and all these organisms starts multiplication so that as time goes on, bacterial count of milk goes on increasing until it is subjected to suitable processing methods.

Bacteria and other microorganisms, utilises the nutrients in milk for their growth and multiplication and deteriorate the quality of milk. Deterioration taking place is not by the depletion of nutrients alone, but mainly due to the accumulation of metabolic wastes, which alter the physicochemical properties of milk and makes it unusable. Deterioration is fast when the bacterial count of milk is high and also when the holding temperature is more. So milk stored at room temperature will get spoiled faster than milk at low temperature. Naturally, keeping quality of milk can be increased by two methods such as reducing the bacterial load in the milk and/or reducing the storage temperature.

Unprocessed raw milk can be stored at room temperature without spoilage for 8-10 hours only. Processing steps should be initiated immediately after milking so nat near original quality of milk can be preserved. Milk intended fr household or local usage purposes can be processed at these places itself immediately after its arrival. However milk sold to large scale collection - distribution systems are usually processed at special processing centres called dairy plants. Here milk from different sources or collection channels are pooled together and collectively processed in large scale processing units. Various operations for increasing keeping quality of milk as described below:

All the precautionary measures described for clean milk production are very important to minimise the bacterial load and thus keeping quality of milk. Again milk is brought in contact with variety of utensils from the production point until reaches before the consumer. These utensils has to be considered as the greatest single source of bacteria and has to be cleaned, sanitised and dried for producing milk with low bacterial count and high keeping quality.

Cleaning and sterilisation of utensils must be done immediately after their use. As the first step rinsing with water is very important in order to remove milk residue. Washing and scrubbing with brush, using plenty of warm water and suitable detergents is very important to remove the residue of milk fat. Sterilising is done by means of hot water or steam or chemicals such as chlorine solution. Steam sterilisation is preferred as it is more effective, removes the residue of detergents and causes immediate drying. Following chemical sterilisation, washing with clean water has to be repeated in order to remove the residue of chemical used and has to be dried by other means.

Production of milk is confined to rural areas in most of the countries, while its demand is more in urban areas. Hence milk has to be collected and transported to processing and distribution points. Collection is usually done by co operative organisations like milk societies or by contractors centred around milk production areas. Milk is then transported by suitable means to near by processing centres. Mode of conveyance varies depending upon the quantity of milk, distance to be transported and collective nature of transportation. If distance is more or there is delay before transporting, cooling/chilling of milk is advised so as to reduce bacterial activity and quality deterioration.

Various processes involved starting from the reception of milk in the dairy plant till the time of its storage for distribution to consumers include:

Filtration/Clarification

It is the process of removing visible foreign particles which have gained entry into the milk. This can be hairs, milk clots, insects, dung particles, soil or dust particles and so on. Filtration involves pouring c f milk through strainers fitted with suitable wire mesh or muslin cloth. Clarification is by subjecting the milk to centrifugation so that centrifugal force causes the foreign particles to sediment, and is done using clarifier.

Standardisation

This is the process of adjusting the fat/SNF content of milk to certain pre-determined level. Adjustment can be either raising or lowering the fat/SNF content and is done adding skim milk (fat removed milk) or cream (fat rich portion) as required. For e.g., For raising SNF, skim milk has to be added into the milk or fat has to be removed to the required level, while for enhancing fat content, cream has to be added into the milk.

Pasteurisation/Sterilisation

it is the process of making the milk free from pathogenic organisms through heating to sufficient temperature for required time. Even after pasteurisation, there can be bacteria which are highly resistant to heat, but which are often harmless. Heating is limited to this level so as to avoid deterioration of milk quality. Sterilisation enables destruction of entire bacteria present in milk including the heat resistant ones so that keeping quality is maximum, but it causes varying degree of denaturation of milk components.

Homogenisation

It is the process of breaking the fat globules present in the milk into smaller ones by forcing the milk through a homogeniser. Purpose of this is to ensure uniform suspension of fat globules throughout the milk and thus to prevent the formation of cream layer (accumulation of fat globules at the top layer of milk).

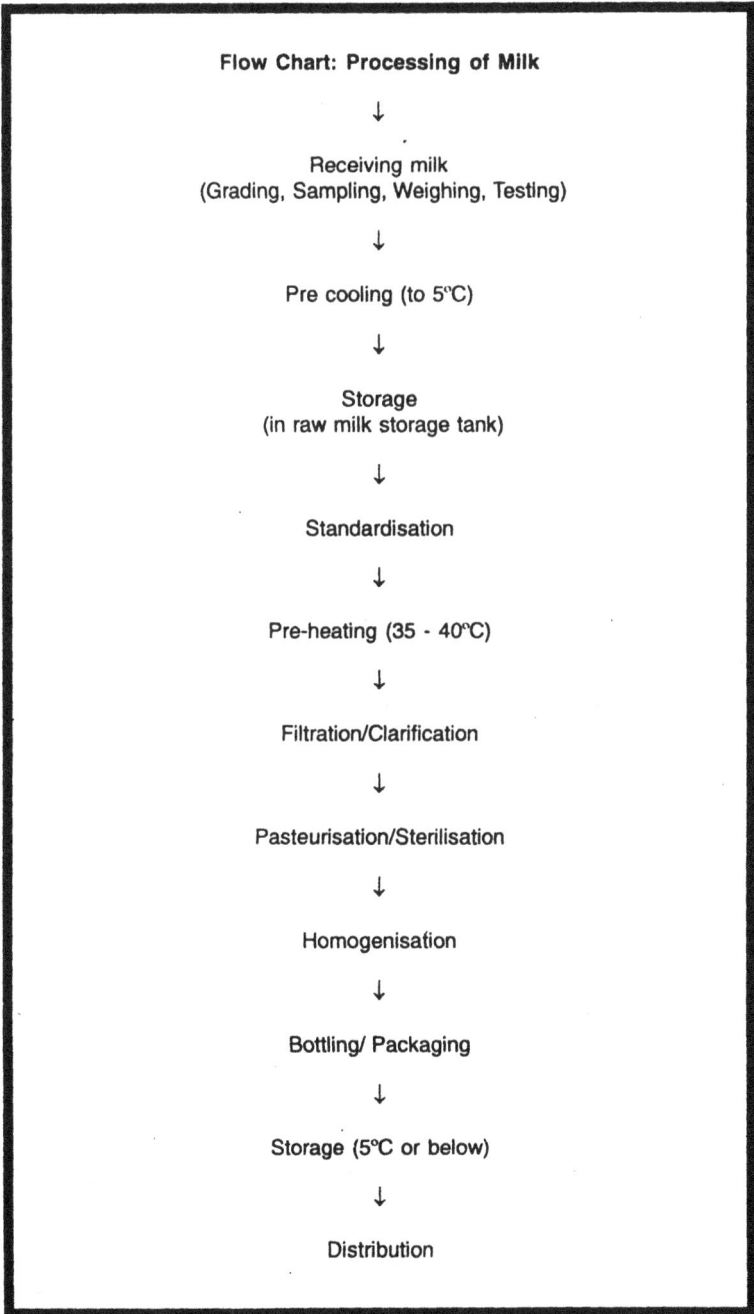

Flow Chart: Processing of Milk

↓

Receiving milk
(Grading, Sampling, Weighing, Testing)

↓

Pre cooling (to 5°C)

↓

Storage
(in raw milk storage tank)

↓

Standardisation

↓

Pre-heating (35 - 40°C)

↓

Filtration/Clarification

↓

Pasteurisation/Sterilisation

↓

Homogenisation

↓

Bottling/ Packaging

↓

Storage (5°C or below)

↓

Distribution

Bottling/Packaging

Bottling/Packaging is done in suitable containers, considering the convenience of storage and distribution. Bottles can be reused after sterilisation, but requires more space and care at handling. Now a days plastic bags are used for packaging so that it is very convenient to use and can be disposed after the use. Thus it is more cheap, but produces disposal problems and pollution. Packages are properly sealed to avoid post pasteurisation contamination and are further cooled to minimise bacterial activity.

Under household conditions, milk is made harmless through boiling for few seconds. Milk is diluted with small quantity of clean water so as to minimise frothing and sticking onto the vessel. Then the vessel is heated with intermittent mixing until boiling for few seconds and is then allowed to cool slowly. By this process every particle of milk will get heated above 85 - 90 °C and allowed to remain at this temperature for few minutes so that pathogenic organisms are destroyed. Milk is then kept closed in suitable bottles either under room temperature or under refrigeration so that it can be preserved upto 8-12 hours (18 -20 hours under refrigeration) without any quality deterioration.

Pasteurisation and Sterilisation

Raw milk received at the dairy is stored in raw milk storage tank after chilling so that its quality deterioration during holding can be minimised. If the milk is found fit for processing based on quality assessment it is subjected to further processing as mentioned earlier.

Pasteurisation is the most common method of processing and is done to render milk safer for human consumption by destroying all pathogenic organisms and to improve keeping quality of milk by reducing bacterial count. At the same time pasteurisation avoids major changes in physico chemical qualities of milk and nutritional value.

The term pasteurisation has been derived from name of the scientist (Louis Pasteur), who invented this technique of processing. He demonstrated that preservation of wine can be done by heating to a temperature of 50 - 60 degree Celsius, and this principle was used for preservation of milk. The term refers to the process of heating every particles of milk to at least 63 °C (145 °F) for 30 minutes or 72 °C

(161 °F) for 15 seconds or to any temperature time combination, which is equally efficient. After pasteurisation, the milk is immediately cooled to 5 °C (41 °F) or below.

The main object of pasteurisation is 1) to render the milk safer for human consumption by destruction of all pathogenic microorganisms 2) to improve the keeping quality of milk by destroying almost all organisms (85 to 99%). The temperature time combination should be such that it should be able to destroy the organisms responsible for TB (Tuberculosis), since these organisms are considered most heat resistant among the pathogenic organisms commonly seen in milk. The phosphatase enzyme present in milk should get inactivated through pasteurisation. So content of this enzyme present in milk is considered as an index for detecting inadequate pasteurisation.

Methods of Pasteurisation

Different methods are used depending upon how the process is carried out as well as the temperature - time combination employed. Commonly adopted methods include:

1. High temperature - short time pasteurisation (HTST) process
2. Batch/holding Pasteurisation and
3. In bottle pasteurisation

High Temperature-Short Time (HTST) Pasteurisation

This was first developed by APV company in the UK in 1922. It is the modern method of pasteurisation and is invariably used where large volume of milk is to be handled. The HTST pasteuriser gives a continuous flow of milk, which is heated to 72 °C for 15 seconds and promptly cooled to 5 °C or below. Milk flows through various stages continuously such as balance tank, pump, regenerative heating, holding, regenerative cooling and cooling by chilled water. Arrangement for incorporation of filter/clarifier, homogeniser etc is also provided in the circuit when designed. There are some variations in the use or order of these steps in different milk processing plants.

HTST pasteuriser has plate type heat exchangers arranged as sequential compartments. Raw milk entering at one end flows continuously by gravity through all the chambers and various steps such as heating and cooling are completed by the time it reaches the other end of pasteuriser. Chilled milk entering the pasteuriser is first pre heated to 35 - 40 ° C in a heat regeneration compartment by the counter flow of hot milk on other side of heat exchanger. Pre heated milk passes through a filter for removing particulate matter if any, and pre heating helps easy flow through the filter.

Milk is then subjected to required level of heating in another set of plate type heat exchangers again by counter flow hot water. Heated milk then goes to a holding section, where the milk is held hot for the required time as specified. From here milk goes via a flow diversion valve, which diverts the flow either back to heating section or into another regenerative cooling section. If the milk is not sufficiently heated it is taken to a balancing tank where from it repeats all the above steps. While properly heated milk is cooled in another set of heat exchangers by the counter flows of chilled raw milk and further by chilled water. Chilled milk thus emerging out goes to pasteurised milk storage tank or packaging/bottling section.

Standard of pasteurisation is judged based on:

Bacterial Destruction
All pathogenic organisms should have destroyed. Tuberculosis bacteria are considered most heat resistant among pathogenic organisms and pasteurisation should be effective to destroy these organisms and is used as an index of pasteurisation efficacy. If TB organisms are destroyed, all other pathogenic organisms also might have destroyed.

Cream Line Reduction
Cream line gives indication of heating time as the same progressively decreases by the temperature and time of heating and consumers uses this criterion for judging quality.

Enzyme Inactivation
Complete destruction of Phosphatase enzyme is useful as a measure for adequacy of pasteurisation process.

Thus optimum pasteurisation ensures complete destruction of pathogens, negative test for phosphatase and least damage to cream line. Major advantages of HTST Pasteurisation:

1. Being a continuous process, there is no wastage of time, material and labour. Milk can be bottled within few minutes of entering the plant

2. Very less space is required when compared to other types of pasteurisers

3. Low initial investment is sufficient to set up a comparatively larger unit

4. Maximum use of regenerative heating and cooling reduces cost of operation

5. Equipment is easily cleaned and sterilised since C.I.P. cleaning is possible

6. Contamination from out side is minimum since it is continuous and closed

7. Possibility of handling even 10 % more milk above the specified capacity.

There are some disadvantages as well such as:

1. Not useful for handling small quantities and other liquid milk products

2. Gasket require constant attention for possible damage and lack of sanitation

3. There will be formation of a narrow cream line and even accumulation of milk stones

Batch/Holding Pasteurisation

Other than HTST method, common method for pasteurisation of milk is Batch/Holding pasteurisation. This is also called as low temperature long time (LTLT) method. The milk is heated to 63 °C or 145 °F for 30 minutes and is then promptly cooled to 5 °C or below. In this system heating is done indirectly, wherein the heat moves through a metal wall in to the product for heating and out of the product for cooling. Batch or holding pasteuriser can be of three types such as:

Water Jacketed Vat

This contains a vessel, which is double walled around the sides and bottom, in which hot water or steam under partial vacuum circulates for heating and subsequently cold water for cooling. Outer wall is usually insulated to reduce heat loss and heat exchange takes place through inner wall. Milk in the vat is agitated slowly by means of propellers. During heating the vat is kept open to allow escape of off flavours. After heating to required temperature, required holding time is allowed during which an air space or foam heater enables to maintain the temperature at the pasteurisation level. Advantages of this type of pasteuriser is flexibility of usage for different milk volumes and products (multi purpose vat)

Water Spray Type

A film of water is sprayed from a perforated pipe against the side walls of the inner tank holding the milk. Milk in the tank is agitated and a rapidly moving continuous film of water provides rapid heat transfer. It is also flexible in usage as in the case of water-jacketed vat.

Coil Vat Type

The heating or cooling medium is pumped through a coil placed either horizontally or vertically, at the same time coil also rotates through the milk so that both heat transfer and agitation take place simultaneously. Disadvantage is difficulty of cleaning the coil.

In Bottle Pasteurisation

This is another method of pasteurisation, wherein bottles filled with raw milk and tightly sealed with special caps are heated to 63-65 °C (145 - 150 °F) for 30 minutes. Then bottles pass through water sprays of decreasing temperatures, which cool the bottle and milk inside. In this method possibility of post - pasteurisation contamination is minimum, while the disadvantages includes slow heat transfer, possibility of bottle breakage, larger bottles has to be used to allow milk expansion during heating and special types of water tight caps has to be used.

Sterilisation

It is another type of processing of milk and refers to the process of heating milk continuously to a temperature of 115 °C for 15 minutes or 145 °C for 3 seconds or equivalent time temperature combination, to ensure preservation of milk at room temperature for a period not less than 15days. As in the case of pasteurisation, sterilisation also can be done in different ways such as:

In Bottle Sterilisation

Here milk is filled and tightly sealed in pre-sterilised bottles. These bottles are then placed in metal crates and placed into the steriliser for heating to 115 °C for 30 minutes. After heat treatment, the milk bottles may be cooled in air or water. This method is simple and flexible, but for large scale processing this method cannot be used for economic reasons. This method also causes a brownish appearance and cooked taste to milk.

Ultra High Temperature Short Time Method (UHT Method)

In this process the milk is heated to 135 - 150 °C for a few seconds generally in a plate or tubular type heat exchanger. As the milk is sterilised in a continuous flow steriliser, large volume of milk can be handled. The milk thus sterilised is almost sterile and is filled in suitable containers for distribution. The filling in containers has to be done aseptically for longer shelf life. Here appearance and taste of milk are not much affected compared to in bottle sterilisation.

Sterilised milk being popularised now a days for various advantages such as:

1. Remarkable keeping quality without need for refrigeration
2. No cream plug formation hence pleasing appearance to buyers
3. Suitable for feeding patients due to formation of easily digestible soft curd
4. Safe for feeding infants since bacteria free and easily digestible
5. Distinctive rich flavour due to homogenisation and less liable to develop oxidised taint.

Main disadvantages include increased cost of production, more loss of nutrients than in pasteurisation and thus reduced biological value.

Bottling/Packaging

After pasteurisation/sterilisation and cooling milk is promptly packaged or bottled before further contamination, loss, damage or degradation due to micro organisms or insects. A package must perform the three fold functions of containing, protecting and merchandising.

Bottling is the traditional method and is still widely used. Bottling when quantity to be handled is more, done mechanically using continuous bottle filling machines, which can be gravity type or vacuum fillers. Vacuum fillers have the advantage that broken bottles are not filled and enable automatic discarding of such bottles. Milk from the cooler goes directly onto the filling machine. Usually bottle-washing operations are so timed along with milk processing that bottles will be ready for immediate filling when processing is completed. Modern mechanical fillers also have the provision for checking the cleanliness of bottles before filling. If any dirt is detected such bottle are rejected automatically..

Caps and Capping

Filling has to be followed by capping and is also mechanically synchronised with filling operation. Cap functions to retain the milk inside the bottle, protects from contamination and seal bottles against tampering. Different types of caps are available and aluminium foil type of caps are commonly used. Capped bottles are then moved automatically into a crater and in between presence and intactness caps are checked again automatically. Dirty bottles are fed back to bottle washer and dirty crates are washed at crate washer before reusing.

Packaging in single service paper or plastic containers is widely used now a days for retail distribution of milk. Most popular type is sachets, which are flexible water- proof bags. Sachet filling is done automatically and filling is followed by a sealing system. Sachets are formed from reeled films, which are continuous. Formed sachets are immediately filled from time-regulated valves, heat sealed and then cut and removed to form individual sachets with milk. Advantages of paper / film package over glass bottles are:

1. Light in weight, easy to handle and less danger of breakage
2. Less distribution cost since less space and labour is required
3. Since no reuse, collection and washing costs are avoided
4. Tamper proof and creates less noise and danger at handling

5. Effective printing of sales message is possible

6. Filling machinery is compact and requires less space

7. No container deposit is needed for distribution through agencies.

Disadvantages

1. High cost per unit of milk distributed

2. Difficult to remove cream

3. Regular supply of film is essential

4. Some cases of leakage may happen

Storage and Distribution

In any dairy plants, processed milk has to be stored for some time. Hence there requires refrigerated rooms where milk can be stored until delivery. Storage of milk in these rooms below 5 °C minimise bacterial growth and prolongs storage life. Distribution is the final stage of market milk industry. For wide distribution it should be properly planned and executed. Distribution requires physical equipments and personnel for transporting the product from the storage area to the consumer or retailers and sales promotion personnel. Besides all these, quality of product, attractive packaging, neat and courteous route salesman, delivery equipments of pleasing appearance, efficient use of men and equipments and effective advertising, decide success of distribution.

Marketing Defects in Milk

Consumer's acceptability of a dairy product depends upon its organoleptic qualities such as appearance, feeling, smell, taste, etc., which the consumer experiences when the product is tasted or consumed. In order to check the acceptability of milk units intended for distribution, samples may be taken and the following observations may be carried out.

1. Closure should be carefully observed and scored

2. Glass bottles should be observed for fullness, cleanliness and freedom from leakage

3. Sample package is then opened and examined for any abnormality of flavour

4. Temperature should be around 16-21°C or 60-70 °F
5. Milk is then examined for the presence of sediment
6. Lastly bacterial count has to be assessed by standard plate count.

Flavour is the single item carrying maximum importance in deciding consumers' acceptability. Hence it is desirable to know the flavour defects, their causes and means of prevention.

Chapter 14
SPECIAL MILKS

Special milks include those processed or fermented milk products, which practically resemble and behave like liquid milk. This includes:

Standardised Milk

It is the milk in which fat and SNF have been adjusted to certain pre-determined levels. Standardisation is usually done mixing raw milk with freshly reconstituted skim milk in proper proportions. As per PFA rules (1976), the standardised milk for liquid consumption should contain a minimum of 4.5 % fat and 8.5 % SNF through out the country. It can be cow milk or buffalo milk or a combination of both in which fat and SNF are adjusted to above levels by extraction or addition of milk fat and /or skim milk or by addition of recombined or reconstituted skimmed milk. Standardised milk shall be pasteurised and shall show a negative phosphatase test.

Advantages of standardised milk are:

1. Ensures practically uniform and constant composition and nutritive value
2. Surplus fat obtained can be converted into butter and ghee
3. Possible to supply milk at comparatively cheaper rates
4. More easily digestible due to low fat content

Toned Milk

It is obtained by mixing water, skim milk powder and whole

milk together to produce milk with 3 % fat. Under PFA rules (1976) toned milk should contain 3 % fat and 8.5 % SNF throughout the country. Usually it is manufactured by admixing high fat milk with skim milk reconstituted out of spray dried skim milk powder. It shall be ensured that the product remains homogenous and no deposition of solids takes place on standing. Also it is mandatory that toned milk should be properly labelled for information of the consumers.

Advantages of toned milk are:

1. Increases supply and thus availability of milk to more people
2. Reduces price of milk so as to reach the lower income groups
3. Can be produced more economically especially if buffalo milk is used

Double Toned Milk

It is similar to toned milk except that it contains less fat content. Under PFA rules (1976) double-toned milk should contain a minimum of 1.5 % fat and 9 % SNF. Advantages and method of manufacture are similar to that of toned milk.

Homogenised Milk

It is the milk treated such a way to ensure break up of fat globules to such an extend that even after 48 hours of storage, no visible cream separation occurs on the milk and fat % does not vary by more than 10 % between top and bottom levels of milk stored in bottle. In efficiently homogenised milk fat globules are sub divided to a size of 2 microns or less diameter. It is done forcing the milk through a homogeniser so as to break the fat globules and is usually done at a temperature above the melting point of fat for easy breakage. Sequences of operations in manufacture are pre-heating, homogenisation, clarification, pasteurisation and cooling.

Advantages are:

1. Avoids cream plug formation stabilising milk fat emulsion
2. Avoids churning of fat through excessive agitation or rough handling
3. Enables easier dispensing of milk since no mixing needed in between

4. More palatable due to brighter appearance, more viscosity and rich flavour

5. Produces easily digestible soft curd, hence better for infant feeding

Major disadvantages are:

1. Increased cost of production

2. More chance for appearance of sediment upon standing

3. Difficulty of fat recovery from packets returned from distribution

4. More susceptible to develop activated sunshine flavour defect

Reconstituted Milk

This refers to milk prepared by dispersing whole milk powder in water to get almost similar composition as that of milk. Since the proportion of solids in milk is approximately 1:7, one part of milk powder is dispersed in 7 part of water so that the properties will be similar to that of whole milk, provided the powder used is whole milk powder and not skim milk powder. Spray dried powder is used commonly since it is more soluble and produce less sediments. Manufacturing is done along with pasteurisation by mixing spray dried whole milk powder with hot water (38 - 43 °C) in a special powder mixer. The mixture is then pumped through a filter into the pasteuriser. Major advantage is that shortage of milk supply in developing countries can be made up adequately.

Recombined Milk

This is the milk obtained by mixing butter oil with skim milk powder and water in suitable proportion. Suitable mechanical treatments are necessary to mix these items properly. This process is usually adopted in dairies to make up the milk deficit during lean season. Under PFA rules (1976) it should contain not less than 3 % fat and 8.5 % SNF. Dried skim milk is reconstituted with water and melted fat is emulsified into it passing through a homogeniser. Recombined milk was extensively produced under Operation flood programme in India. Major advantages are:

1. Shortage of fresh milk supply in developing countries can be made up
2. Helps in stabilising the price of milk in cities.

Filled Milk

This resembles recombined milk but vegetable fats are used in place of butter fat.

Condensed Milk

Condensed milk is a product obtained by evaporating part of water from whole milk or from fully or partly skimmed milk, with or without addition of any sugar. Condensed milk sweetened by sugar and added with some flavour is usually called flavoured milk, while non-sweetened condensed milk is called evaporated milk, which is not very popular.

Flavoured Milk

Flavoured milk are milk products containing milk added with flavouring agents. Edible flavours such as chocolate, coffee, rose, etc. are added to pasteurised or sterilised milk along with edible colours and cane sugar. When the term milk is used on the label, the product should contain a milk fat percentage legally required for market milk. When fat is lower than that, the term drink is used. Advantage is that milk is made more palatable to those who do not relish it as such and skim milk is put to profitable usage.

Common types of flavoured milk are:

1. Chocolate milks/drinks
2. Fruit flavoured milks/drinks
3. Sterilised flavoured milks/drinks.

Manufacturing of Chocolate Milk

Ingredients required

1. Cocoa powder 1 - 1.5 %,
2. Sugar 5 to 7 %
3. Stabiliser 0.2 %
4. Milk having minimum fat level as per legal standard.

Cocoa powder is to give flavour and stabiliser prevents settling of cocoa particles and to minimise cream rising. The milk is standardised, pre heated (60 °C) and homogenised. To the warm milk add desired amounts of cocoa, sugar and stabiliser slowly and with stirring. The milk is then pasteurised, cooled, bottled and stored under refrigeration.

Fruit flavoured milk is prepared by adding permitted fruit flavours and colours instead of cocoa powder and other steps in manufacture are the same. No acids should be added to fruit flavour as it may cause curdling. Fruit flavour is added at the rate of 1 part to every 5 parts of milk.

Sterilised flavoured milk is prepared in the same way as that of sterilised milk except for the addition of suitable flavour, colour and sugar before sterilisation.

Cultured milk refers to those milks, which have been made by employing selected micro organisms to develop characteristic flavour and / or body and texture. Culture is the term used to refer an active bacterial culture that has been propagated for use in the manufacture of fermented milk or milk products. Active culture performs three important functions in the manufacture of fermented products such as:

1. Acid production
2. Production of desired flavour and
3. Prevention of the growth of undesirable microorganisms that might have survived pasteurisation or entered as contaminants.

Examples of cultured milk are Acidophilus milk, Bulgarian milk, Kumis, Kefir etc.

Vitaminised or Irradiated Milk

It is milk to which one or more vitamins are added. Irradiated milk is one in which Vitamin D content is increased by exposure to U.V. light

Humanised Milk

Cow milk or buffalo milk made to resemble chemical composition of human milk is called humanised milk

Soft Curd Milk

It is milk that forms a soft curd when coagulated with rennet under standard procedures. It is characterised by low casein and calcium content. Mother's milk is best for feeding infants since it forms a soft curd when coagulated in the stomach and is more quickly digested by infants.

Vegetable Toned Milk

It is the milk in which milk protein is substituted by vegetable protein isolated from ground nut

Imitation Milk

A product resembling milk but of non dairy origin

Chapter 15
COMMON MILK PRODUCTS

Milk is used for human consumption in the form of milk as such, or as an ingredient of different food items or in the form of various products. Purpose of converting milk into its products can be:

Improves Keeping Quality of Milk

Milk being highly perishable, it needs processing to increase its keeping quality and even then its shelf life is affected by storage conditions. However shelf life of milk can be extended considerably through conversion into different milk products.

Minimises Storage Facilities

For better shelf life of processed milk, there is need for refrigeration, however milk products can be stored at room temperature for very long time.

Less Storage Space

Major proportion of milk being water, storage of milk as such requires lot of space, however conversion of milk into solid products considerably reduces the storage space requirement.

Avoids Marketing Problems

Raw milk has to be disposed without further delay so as to minimise quality deterioration and there is need for ready marketing. However conversion into products avoids the urgency of marketing and need for ready market.

Utilisation of Seasonal Surplus

During flood season, there will be large volume of milk, which often cannot be marketed. Such surplus milk can be converted into products for better utilisation and increased return.

Possibility of Reconstitution

Milk converted into milk powder during surplus season can be reconstituted back into milk in order to make up the seasonal shortages in supply.

Solves the Problems of Unforeseen Market Failures

Milk otherwise wasted due to unforeseen transport or market interruptions can be utilised through preparation of products.

Better Nutritive Value

Some of the products are better digested than milk and have better nutritive as well as medicinal value due to the processes taking place during the formation of milk products

Preference

Milk products are liked by even those people not taking raw milk for dislike or diseases like allergy and digestive problems

Diversification

Milk products allows to make variety dishes for parties and also enables better marketing through product diversification.

Employment

Milk product units provides more employment opportunities in villages especially to women and elderly

Enables Export

While exporting raw milk is cumbersome, milk products can be easily exported earning foreign money.

There are many types of popular milk products, which are prepared either at home or as small scale or larger scale industrial units. Types of product prevalent in an area depend on many factors such as quantity of milk available, traditional practices, dietary habits of people, market demand, purchasing power of people and other local conditions. The products can be broadly classified into some groups based on the method of manufacture such as fermented, frozen, separated, concentrated, coagulated and dried products.

Fermented Products

Fermented products are prepared by subjecting the milk to fermentation by certain types of bacteria. Fermentation has been defined as metabolic process in which chemical changes are brought about on an organic substrate such as protein, carbohydrate or fat through the action of microorganisms. Microorganisms thus introduced multiply utilising the components of milk and produce various metabolic by products and end products, which in turn impart characteristic flavour and consistency to the milk. Depending upon the type of organisms involved in fermentation, organoleptic quality and nutritive value of the resultant product varies.

Normal fermentation of milk is lactic acid fermentation, which is the process by which lactic acid is produced under the usual conditions of fermentation. Abnormal fermentations are those that cause other changes such as sweet curdling, ropiness, gas, colour, flavour etc on account of microorganisms.

Starter Culture

Specific types of bacteria added to milk for getting desired type of fermentation is called starter culture. The term refers to an active bacterial culture that has been propagated for use in the manufacture of fermented milk products. Lactic starter usually indicates a culture containing lactic streptococci. Starter species most commonly used are *Streptococcus lactis, S. cremoris, S. diacetyl lactis* and *Leuconostoc sp.* Functions of starter includes acid production, desired characteristic flavour production and prevention of growth of undesirable microorganisms that may have survived the pasteurisation or contaminated the product.

Propagation of Starter

Each fermented milk product requires selected starter culture in its manufacture. Commercial starter cultures are prepared by commercial laboratories and are available in liquid, tablet or powder forms; they may be freeze-dried as well. Propagation of starter includes steps such as propagation of mother culture, intermediate culture and bulk starter.

Mother culture refers to stock lactic cultures prepared routinely in the dairy plant for day to day bulk propagation. For preparing mother couture the milk should be of high quality, low microbial count and free of inhibitory substances. This milk is taken in a clean sterile glass bottle (1 quart capacity), heated to 82 °C for 1 hour and cooled to 20-22 °C for inoculation. Previous days mother starter is added at the rate of 1 % under aseptic conditions. The contents are mixed well and incubated at 22 °C for 14 - 16 hours until an acidity of 0.75 to 0.85 % is developed. It is then cooled to 5 °C and stored in refrigerator.

Intermediate culture: This is prepared when more quantity of mother culture is needed for inoculating milk in large bulk tanks. Normally intermediate culture is prepared in glass bottles of 4 - 20 litres size.

Bulk starter refers to the starter made in large amounts whenever required for the manufacture of fermented milk or its products. The preparation of starter culture in larger volume presents difficulties in preventing contamination. For preparing bulk starter, milk is heated to 85-90 °C for 45 - 60 minutes and cooled rapidly to the inoculation temperature of 22 °C. The bulk milk is then inoculated immediately with 1 % inoculum from a fresh mother culture. For convenience an intermediate culture is prepared for inoculating the bulk. After inoculation the contents are mixed properly and allowed to ferment at 22 °C for 14 - 16 hours till an acidity of 0.75 to 0.85 % is reached and the starter is rapidly cooled to 5 °C and stored in refrigeration for use.

Starter Qualities

Usual flavours of starter culture are mild, pleasant nutty smell and clean acid taste. Body of starter should be soft and firm. Curd should give clean and smooth break without any gas holes. Texture should be smooth and free from lumps. Titratable acidity should be 0.75 to 0.85 %. Starter defects include insufficient flavour development, insufficient acid development, hard and lumpy curd, excessive development of acidity, gas holes, ropiness, bitterness, presence of bacteriophage etc.

Curd (Dahi)

It is the most commonly used fermented milk product. Indian curd is also called Dahi and is consumed by a large section of population throughout the country. It has been established that the food and nutritive value of dahi is more than that of original milk since it is more palatable, digestible and assimilated than milk. Also it has been said that dahi has got some therapeutic value for some stomach and intestinal disorders, possibly due to its content of antibiotic substances. Dahi can be classified into two types 1) Dahi for churning into desi butter and Dahi for direct consumption.

According to PFA rules(1976) Dahi or curd is the product obtained from pasteurised or boiled milk by souring naturally or otherwise by a harmless lactic acid or other bacterial culture. It should have same percentage of fat and SNF as the milk from which it is prepared.

Method of Preparation

Prepared by fermentation of milk adding suitable starter culture. Milk is boiled and cooled to room temperature and then inoculated with 0.5 to 1 % starter culture (previous days Dahi or butter milk) and allowed to remain overnight without any disturbance. By the time bacteria present in the starter (lactic acid bacteria such as Streptococcus and Lactobacillus species) will ferment the lactose in milk and produces lactic acid. The lactic acid content in dahi varies from 0.5 to 1.1 % depending upon the type of starter used and the incubation period. Good quality dahi should appear with smooth glassy surface, mild pleasant smell and clean acid taste.

The lactic acid content in dahi varies from 0.5 to 1.1 % depending upon the type of starter used, incubation period and temperature of incubation. In addition to lactic acid, certain bacteria ferments citrate present in milk and is responsible for the typical flavour of curd. There should be an optimum proportion of acid producing and flavour producing bacteria to obtain the normal qualities of dahi. Good quality dahi should appear with smooth glassy surface, mild pleasant smell and clean acid taste. Sometime bacterial contaminants in milk cause certain undesirable types of fermentation leading to gas production, whey separation and so on.

Lassi

It refers to Desi butter milk obtained during production of Makhan or Desi butter. It contains appreciable amount of milk proteins and phospholipids. Lassi is used as a:

1. Beverage (by adding sugar or salt with or without additional flavours. *E.g.*, "Sambaram"
2. Starter culture
3. Coagulant etc.

Beaten whole milk curd with added sugar is also called Lassi in certain regions.

Yoghurt

Yoghurt is a fermented product similar to dahi prepared from milk of high solid content. It is a common milk product in Bulgaria and gaining popularity in India and other countries as well. Some quantity of water is evaporated from milk or skim milk powder is added. This milk of high SNF content is then subjected to fermentation by the symbiotic growth of two types of bacteria (*Lactobacillus bulgaricus and Streptococcus thermophilus*). The resultant product is quite thicker than dahi and is usually used for direct consumption with or without sweetening by addition of sugar.

Chapter 16
FAT RICH PRODUCTS

Cream

Fat rich portion separated from whole milk is called cream. It contains all the milk constituents in varying proportions. The milk fat in cream may vary from 18 to 85 % and SNF constituents occur in lower proportion than in milk. According to PFA rules (1976) cream should contain a minimum of 25 % milk fat. Depending upon fat % and mode of usage cream can be of different types such as table cream, light cream, coffee cream and all these contains 20-25 % milk fat. Whipping cream and heavy cream contains 30-49% fat. Plastic cream contains 65-85% milk fat.

Methods of Cream Separation

Cream separation is done by two methods such as gravity and centrifugal methods. The basic principle of cream separation by either of the methods is the density difference between fat and skim milk portion. At 16 °C (60 °F) the average density of milk fat is 0.93 and that of skim milk is 1.036. Fat being lighter than skim milk, it raises to the top of the skim milk layer.

Milk is a mixture of fat and skim milk, which when subjected to either gravity or centrifugal force, the two components by virtue of their density difference separate from one another. In gravity method, when milk is allowed to stand for some time there is a tendency for the fat to rise to the top of the vessel. This method being very slow, no longer used for commercial purpose.

Instrument used for separating cream based on the principle of centrifugal force is known as centrifugal cream separators. Cream separators consists of number of conical disks arranged one over another so that these disks rotates with a high speed. Centrifugal force thus subjected to milk is 3000 - 6000 times greater than gravitational force. When milk is distributed over these disks, the skim milk portion (heavier portion) moves towards periphery, while the fat portion moves towards the centre of the cream separator, thus enabling their separation.

Factors affecting fat % of cream during centrifugal separation includes:

Position of Cream Screw or Skim Milk Screw

Cream screw or out let consists of a small threaded hollow screw pierced by circular orifice through which the cream emerges. This screw can be driven IN or OUT thus bringing it nearer to or away from the centre of rotation. Similarly the skim milk screw is for the removal of skim milk. Once the cream screw or skim milk screw has been adjusted, the cream separator delivers cream and skim milk at a definite ratio. By altering the position of cream screw or skim milk screw, the ratio of skim milk to cream changes. Thus when the cream screw is moved in, or skim milk screw out a higher fat % cream is obtained and vice versa.

Fat % in Milk

Higher the fat % in milk higher the fat % in cream and vice versa.

Speed of Separator

Higher the speed, higher the fat % in cream and vice versa

Rate of Milk Inflow

Higher the rate of milk inflow, lower the fat % in cream and vice versa

Temperature of Milk

Lower the temperature of milk during cream separation, higher the percentage of fat in cream and vice versa.

Amount of Water or Skim Milk Added to Flush the Separator

Greater the quantity of water or skim milk added to flush the separator, lower the fat % in cream and vice versa.

Processing of Cream

Cream is subjected to different types of processing depending upon the desired quality of the final product.

Neutralisation of Cream

Neutralisation of sour cream for butter making refers to a partial reduction of its acidity. The acidity of freshly separated cream is always lower than that of milk from which it was separated. During storage its acidity increases. Normally neutralisation is done for high acid cream during butter making. Usage of high acid cream for butter making will result in excessive fat loss in buttermilk and production of undesirable flavour in butter. Cream for making butter intended for long storage should have 0.06 to 0.08 % acidity and that for early consumption should be 0.25 to 0.3 %.

There are two types of neutralisers available for use such as lime (Calcium hydroxide and Magnesium hydroxide) and soda (caustic soda or sodium hydroxide and sodium bicarbonate). The amount of neutraliser added depends upon acidity of cream, final acidity of butter desired and type of neutraliser compound used.

Standardisation of Cream

This refers to the adjustment of fat level in cream to the desired level. The fat % in cream is usually lowered to the prescribed level by the addition of a calculated amount of skim milk and is increased by re separating the low fat cream.

Pasteurisation of cream

Same as for milk

Packaging and Storage

Table cream is packaged for retail sale in units similar to those for milk such as glass bottles, paper carton, Polythene sachets, plastic bottles etc. Storage of cream is preferably done at 5-10 °C.

Uses of Cream

Cream is mainly used for the production of butter and ghee. Other uses include preparation of some special dishes, ice cream and direct consumption as coffee whiteners.

Butter

Butter is the concentrated form of milk fat collected by churning either cream or dahi. According to PFA rules (1976), butter should contain not less than 80 % fat (Desi-butter - 76 %), a maximum of 1.5 % curd content and a maximum of 3 % common salt. Since butter is very high in fat, it contains all the fat soluble vitamins such as Vitamin A, D, E and K. Types of butter commonly made such as Pasteurised cream butter, ripened or un-ripened butter, salted or unsalted butter, sweet cream butter or sour cream butter, fresh butter or cold stored butter, Dairy butter or creamery butter.

Method of Preparation

In households, Makhan (desi - butter) is made by churning dahi using crude indigenous devices. Commercially butter manufacturing is done from cream through churning process using large/ commercial butter churns. Normally cream having 35-40 % fat is used. Cream can be un-ripened (fresh) or ripened cream (cream subjected to fermentation with the help of desirable starter culture). Ripened cream produces a pleasant flavour and also reduces fat loss in butter milk.

Before feeding into the butter churn, cream is cooled to 5-10 °C and held overnight at this temperature and this process is called as ageing of cream. Ageing is done to make partial solidification of fat globules so that churning becomes easier. The quantity of cream fed into the butter churn is usually 1/3 to ½ the capacity of churn. After feeding cream, the churn is rotated either manually or mechanically and the process is called churning.

During churning process agitation of cream occurs and the fat in skim milk emulsion breaks causing adhering of fat globules. As the process continues, more and more fat globules joins together to form larger and larger masses until relatively complete separation of fat and skim milk occurs. At this stage churning is stopped and buttermilk is drained off through a sieve. To ensure complete removal of buttermilk, butter in the churn is washed with chilled water (5 °C). For this chilled water is added into the churn after draining of buttermilk and churning is repeated for few more rotations. Wash water is then drained out and washing is repeated if needed.

If salted butter is to be prepared, common salt is added at the rate of 2 - 2.5 %. Butter is then kneaded by churning for few more revolutions and this process is known as "working" of butter. Working is done to expel the remaining buttermilk inside the butter and thus to bring the butter grains together into a compact mass. Working also helps to dissolve and distribute uniformly the salt throughout the butter. Then the butter is taken out of the churn and stored.

Butter is usually packed in parchment paper (butter paper) or in aluminium foil and stored under refrigeration. Long term storage is usually done at a temperature of -23 to -29 °C. At home in the absence of refrigerator butter is stored in water kept in an earthern pot or in brine solution. In case of storage in water, water has to be changed every day, while in case of brine changing is needed only once in a week.

Over Run in Butter

The amount of butter which exceeds the fat % in cream is called over run in butter. It is usually expressed in percentage. Over run is caused by the presence of moisture, curd, salt etc in butter. Maximum obtainable over run is 25 %.

$$\text{Percentage over run} = \frac{\text{Butter made in Kgs - Fat in churn in Kg}}{\text{Fat in churn in Kgs}} \times 100$$

Salted butter can be used for direct consumption. Unsalted butter is used for the production of ghee, butter oil, ice cream, other dishes and confectionaries. Also used as a cooking medium.

Ghee

It is an important milk product which has been extensively used throughout the country for dietary as well as religious purposes. Ghee is the clarified butter fat prepared either from cream or butter. It is the richest source of milk fat among all dairy products.

Composition

Ghee usually contains:

Table 24

Milk fat	99 - 99.5 %
Moisture	not more than 0.5 %,
Unsaponifiable matter	
Carotene	3.2 - 7.5 microgram / gram
Vitamin A	19 - 34 IU/g
Tocoferrol	26-48 microgram / gram
Free fatty acids	maximum 2.8 % of Oleic acid

Physicochemical Constituents

Ghee, as in the case of other fats and oils, is characterised by certain physicochemical properties. These properties have been found to be the basis of fixation of certain analytical constants for defining the quality of ghee. Some of the important physicochemical constants and their respective value for ghee are:

Melting Point
28 - 40 °C

Solidifying Pint
15 - 28 °C

Specific Gravity
0.93 - 0.94

Refractive Index
At 40 °C BR (Butyro - refracto metre) reading varies from 40 - 45.

RM (Reichert- meissl) Value
This is a measure of volatile soluble fatty acids. It should not be less than 28 except for ghee from cotton seed feeding areas, where the limit is 21

Polenske Value
This is a measure of volatile insoluble fatty acids and normal value of this should not be more than 2

Saponification Value
This is a measure of saponifiable matter in ghee and the normal value should not be less than 220

Iodine Value

This is a measure of degree of unsaturation and the value varies between 26 - 38

PFA standard for Ghee (in Kerala) are the following:

Table 25

BR reading	(at 40 °C)	40 - 43
RM value	(minimum)	26
FFA	(As % of Oleic acid)	3
Moisture	(maximum)	0.3

Method of Preparation

Various methods of preparation of ghee are:

Traditional method (Country/Desi method)

More than 90 % of the ghee is produced in the country by traditional methods such as making desi butter (Makhan) and then converting into ghee. Makhan produced by churning the curd is taken in a metallic vessel and heated with stirring over a low fire to evaporate the moisture. When evaporation is completed, further heating is stopped and the vessel is allowed to cool. After the residue has settled down, the clear fat is poured into suitable containers. In this method the fat recovery is estimated to be 83 %. Also the ghee produced in this method has got very low keeping quality

Modern Methods

Modern methods of ghee making are practised in dairy plants and can be of two types such as:

1. Direct cream method wherein cream is used as the raw material for making ghee
2. *Creamery butter method*: Here creamery butter or butter made in dairy plant is being used.

In both these cases cream or butter is heated in a ghee boiler, which consists of a stainless steel pan provided with a manual stirrer. The pan has got an outlet at the bottom for emptying the contents. Cream or butter is first melted at low heat and the temperature is then increased so that the mass begins to boil. The contents are constantly agitated through out the process to prevent scorching. Usually there will be profuse effervescence, accompanied by a crackling sound during the early stages of boiling, which decrease gradually as the moisture evaporates.

When practically all the moisture has been removed, the temperature of the liquid mass suddenly shoots up, and the heating at this time has to be carefully controlled. The end point is indicated by the appearance of a second effervescence, which is much finer than the first, together with browning of the curd particles. At this stage a characteristic ghee flavour also emenates. The final temperature of ghee at this stage will be 110 - 120 °C. After cooling and sedimentation ghee is filtered through a muslin cloth to remove the sediment known as ghee residue. Direct cream method of ghee making yields higher quantity of ghee residue and takes a long time.

Free Stratification Method

Clarification of butter or cream into ghee by the above methods has certain obvious demerits. In traditional methods there is a much greater possibility of obtaining a finished product characterised by an overheated and smoky flavour. In the creamery method, the high acidity of the raw material at high clarifying temperatures makes the product greasy and also reduces its shelf life. Research work has lead to the evolution of a modified technique capable of yielding a higher grade product at lower cost of clarification.

The principle of this method is as follows. When butter is kept undisturbed at a temperature of 80-85 °C for 15 - 30 minutes, it stratifies into 3 distinct layers, that is a top layer of floating denatured particles of curd, a middle layer of fat and bottom layer of butter milk. This separation into layers has been called as pre-stratification. The bottom layer of buttermilk contains about 60 - 70 % SNF and 80 % of the moisture originally present in butter. The buttermilk is mechanically removed without disturbing the top and middle layers and the temperature of the two layers is raised to the usual clarifying temperature of 110 - 120 °C.

Cooling and Granulation

After clarification ghee is cooled to 1 °C above the melting point of ghee (29 °C) to produce granules in the ghee. This process is called granulation. Indian buyers consider granularity of ghee as an important criterion of quality and even purity. Granulation is due to certain level of glycerides of higher melting point (saturated fatty acids).

The colour of cow ghee is deep yellow, while that of buffalo ghee is white with a characteristic yellowish or greenish tinge. Ghee has a pleasant cooked and rich flavour. The taste is usually characteristic of the milk fat, slightly acidic flavour is sometimes preferred. Ghee is expected to have a storage life of 6- 12 months at 21°C.

Packaging and Storage

Since milk fat is susceptible to deterioration due to exposure to light, air and metals, ghee should be properly packaged promptly after production so as to retain its initial flavour and nutritive value. The commonly used packaging materials include plastic bottles, glass bottles and tin coated cans. The storage temperature of ghee may vary from 5 - 30 °C although refrigerated storage of ghee prolongs its keeping quality, it renders the stored product greasy and pasty. Therefore a storage temperature of 21 °C is usually recommended. Keeping quality of ghee at 21 °C is around 6- 12 months.

Agmark Grading of Ghee

Ghee- the most expensive of edible fats, is adulterated with cheap adulterants by the numerous middle men during production, handling and distribution stages. The main adulterants of ghee are Vanaspati or hydrogenated vegetable oils, refined vegetable oils, animal fats etc. Detection of these adulterants in the household is not much easy, that is the quality as well as purity of ghee can be judged only by detailed physical and chemical analysis. So it is necessary to grade ghee according to its quality and purity. For this purpose, the agmark ghee grading scheme was initiated by the agricultural marketing department.

Under the scheme, recognised ghee dealers can mark ghee in standard container, bearing the seal of Agmark authorities and designating quality of the product. The main objective of agmark grading is to ensure the consumer a product of pre-tested quality and purity. Agmark standard is given only to those ghee, which meet the required standards upon analysis. Agmark ghee is packed under "special" and "General" categories, which are packaged under two differently coloured labels. The only difference in the grades is maximum limit of free fatty acids. For special grade (Red label) ghee, the FFA is limited to 1.4 % and in general grade (green label) it is 2.5%.

Agmark standards for ghee is decided based on the following:

1. *Baudouin test (to detect the presence of Vanaspati in ghee)* : negative

2. *Phytosterol acetate test (to detect the presence of vegetable oils)* : negative

3. *BR reading (At 40 °C)* : 40 - 42

4. *RM value*: Not less than 28

5. *P value*: 1-2

6. *Moisture percentage*: Not more than 0.3

7. *FFA (% oleic) special grade*: Not more than 1.4, General: Not more than 2.5

Butter Oil

Butter oil is another fat concentrated milk product similar to ghee. Butter oil is defined as fat concentrate obtained mainly from butter or cream by the removal of practically all water and solid not fat content. It is prepared by boiling of butter under low pressure so that the fat boils at low temperature and evaporates entire water content. As the evaporation temperature is low, there will be no structural alteration to the fat unlike ghee. Butter oil appears as thick oily substance and is used for making recombined milk.

Composition of butter oil is as follows:

1. Butter fat: 99.5 to 99.8 %

2. Moisture: 0.1 to 0.3 %

3. Acidity (% oleic) : 0.2 - 0.5 %

Chapter 17

COAGULATED AND FROZEN MILK PRODUCTS

Cheese

In India's rapidly expanding dairy industry one product gaining much popularity is cheese. It is one of the oldest foods of mankind. It is a coagulated type of milk product. Cheese contains all the main milk constituents such as protein, fat and minerals in plenty and they are found in cheese in their simpler form. So all the nutrients in cheese are in a readily digestible form.

Cheese has been defined as a product made from milk by coagulating the casein with the help of rennet or similar enzymes in the presence of lactic acid produced by added micro organisms, from which part of moisture has been removed by cutting, cooking and pressing, which has been shaped in mould and then ripened by holding it for sometime at suitable temperature and humidity. According to PFA act hard cheese can have a maximum of 43 % moisture and a minimum of 42 % fat on dry matter basis.

Varieties

At present there are at least 400 cheese varieties. They can be classified based on moisture content, body & texture, curing/ripening and type of ripening etc. For example:

Varieties based on moisture content are:

1. *High moisture cheese varieties*: Cottage cheese, Mozzarella cheese

2. *Medium moisture content*: Cheddar cheese, Swiss cheese

3. *Low moisture*: Parmesan cheese

Based on texture and body:
1. *Hard*: Cheddar cheese
2. *Soft*: Cottage cheese

Based on curing or ripening
1. *Un-ripened*: Cottage
2. *Ripened*: Cheddar

Method of Preparation

Various steps in the preparation of cheese are the following

Receiving Milk

Fresh, filtered milk with good quality is taken in a cheese vat (double jacketed, rectangular vats)

Standardisation

This refers to adjustment of casein/fat ratio in milk to 1: 0.7 to regulate the fat to dry matter of cheese and to ensure cheese of a more uniform composition.

Pasteurisation

72 °C for 15 seconds

Cooling

Cooling to 31 °C

Addition of Calcium Chloride

Excessive heat treatment causes precipitation of a part of calcium salts present in milk. This results in slower Rennet action and a weaker curd, which can be corrected by the addition of 0.01 - 0.03 % calcium chloride to milk.

Addition of Starter

A culture of lactic acid bacteria is added at the rate of 1 % level at 31 °C.

Addition of Rennet

Rennet is added when the milk gets 0.2 % acidity after the addition of starter. Rennet is a milk-coagulating enzyme, which consists mainly pepsin and rennin. Rennet is commercially prepared form the stomach of calves. The amount of rennet added is 2 gram per 100 Kg milk. By adding rennet milk protein is coagulated and complete coagulation occurs within 30 - 60 minutes

Cutting of Curd

For cutting purpose wire knives of both horizontal and vertical types are used. They are called as cheese knives. These knives cut the cheese into ¼ inch cubes

Cooking

It refers to heating of curd cubes from 31 °C to 38 °C at the rate of 1 °C per 5 minutes. During this process the curd particle contract to about half their original size, eliminating considerable water or whey

Drainage of Whey

Whey is removed from the curd by placing a strainer in the vat outlet.

Cheddaring

It refers to the combined operations of packing, block making, turning, piling and re-piling of the curd cubes. When the cheddaring process is completed, the small particles of curd loose their identity fusing together into a practically solid mass of curd. Considerable water or whey is eliminated during this process.

Milling

After cheddaring the curd blocks are passed through a cheese mill, where the blocks of curd are cut into small pieces.

Salting

Salt is added at the rate of 1 % level. It improves the flavour, body and texture and keeping quality of cheese

Hooping

Refers to placing of curd in cheese hoopes or moulds to press the curd into final shape

Pressing

The hooped curd is pressed into its smallest space by placing in a cheese press. Initially small pressure is applied and is increased considerably as the curd packs.

Paraffining

It is the process of dipping curd in a bath of melted paraffin (90 °C) for a few seconds. A thin coating of paraffin wax is formed on the surface of cheese. By this operation all the holes on the cheese surface closes, kills any molds and checks the evaporation of water from cheese during ripening.

Curing

It refers to the storage of cheese for at least 2-3 months at a given low temperature (10 °C) and relative humidity (35 %) during which its physical, chemical and bacteriological properties are changed resulting in the development of characteristic flavour, body and texture. The fat, protein and lactose present in cheese are decomposed into their simpler forms by microbial action

Packaging and Storage

The common forms of packages are tin cans, plastic bags or pouches, glass jars, etc. Cheese is stored at low temperature preferably at 0 - 1 °C to ensure good quality. A high temperature leads to evaporation of moisture, growth of unwanted molds, bacteria etc.

Cottage Cheese

This is a soft un ripened cheese usually made from skim milk. Creamed cottage cheese has cream mixed into it so that the finished product contains not less than 4 % fat. Various steps in the preparation of cottage cheese include

Receiving skim milk - adding calcium chloride - adding starter - Adding rennet - Cutting- cooking - drainage of whey - washing and draining - Salting - creaming - packaging.

Cottage cheese may be packed in wax or polythene coated paper cups or in polythene bags. It should be stored at 5 - 10 °C

Processed Cheese

They are the modified form of natural cheese prepared with the aid of heat, by mixing and blending of one or more lots of cheese with salt, colour, water and emulsifier into a homogenous plastic mass (which is usually packed while hot). It increases the keeping quality.

Uses of Cheese

Used for direct consumption and in the preparation of special dishes and sauses.

Paneer

It is also called chhana in certain parts of the country. It refers to the milk solids obtained by acid coagulation of boiled whole milk and subsequent drainage of whey. If pressure is applied for draining whey, the product is paneer otherwise it is called chhana. The acids commonly used are lactic acid or citric acid. Usual chemical composition of paneer is Moisture 50.7 %, Fat 27.1 %, Protein 17.9 %, Lactose 2.3 % and Minerals 1.8 %. According to PFA standards Paneer should contain not less than 50 % milk fat and moisture content should not exceed 70 %.

Method of Preparation

Milk is heated to near boiling and then coagulated by adding lime juice or 1 % citric acid. After complete coagulation, the coagulated material is taken in a cloth and the liquid portion is drained off. The cooled coagulum is placed in wooden moulds and adequate pressure is applied by putting suitable weight over the mass. The product thus obtained is called paneer. If the cloth containing coagulated material is hung up to drain the whey (without pressing) the : roduct formed is called chhana.

The common packaging materials used are plastic film bags, laminated pouches etc. Paneer stored at room temperature has very low keeping quality. Therefore refrigerated storage is preferred. Keeping quality is influenced by storage temperature, quality of raw milk and moisture content of paneer etc. Keeping quality at 5-10 °C is around 1 week. Paneer can be used for making various milk sweets like Rossogolla, Pantooa, Sandesh, Rasamalai and certain special dishes.

Frozen Milk Products

Ice Cream

It is a frozen dairy product made from suitable blending and processing of cream and other milk products together with sugar and flavour with or without stabiliser or colour and with the incorporation of air during the freezing process. According to PFA standards ice cream should contain:

Table 26

Milk fat	Not less than 10 %
Protein	Not less than 3.5 %
Total solids	Not less than 36 %

Table 27: ISI Specifications for Ice Cream

Weight of 1 litre ice cream	525 grams	Minimum
Total solids	36 %	Minimum
Acidity (in terms of % oleic acid)	0.25	Maximum
Sucrose by weight	15 %	Maximum
Stabiliser / emulsifier by weight	0.5 %	Maximum
SPC per gram	2,50,000	Maximum
Coliform per gram	100	Maximum
Phosphatase test		Negative

Method of Preparation

Various steps include·

Selection of Ingredients

For preparation of ice cream, ice cream mix has to be prepared first. For this various dairy and non-dairy ingredients are selected according to their availability, cost, convenience in handling etc. Commonly selected dairy products are milk and milk products such as:

Table 28

Source of fat	Cream, butte etc
Source of SNF	Skim milk and skim milk powder
Source of both fat and SNF	Whole milk and whole milk powder

Milk and milk products are the source of milk fat and milk SNF, and furnish approximately 60 % of total solids of the ice cream mix. Milk fat enriches and mellows the ice cream giving it a full, rich, creamy flavour. Milk SNF helps to make ice cream compact and smooth.

Non-dairy products selected for ice cream include:

Sweetening Agents

Common sweetening agent used is cane sugar. Main function of sugar is to increase the acceptability of ice cream. Also sugar is the cheapest source of solids in ice cream

Stabilisers

These are used to prevent formation of large ice crystals in ice cream especially during storage. Since they are added in small quantities (0.5 %) they have negligible influence on food value and flavour. Gelatin, sodium alginate and glycerol mono-stearate are examples of the commonly used stabilisers

Emulsifiers

They are mainly used to improve the whipping quality of ice cream mix during freezing. Eg: Egg yolk, Lecithin etc

Flavour and Colour

Flavour increases the acceptability of ice cream. Most popular flavours are Vanilla, chocolate etc. Colour is used for better appearance of ice cream

Figuring of Mix

This is a process of calculating the amount of each ingredient to be used for obtaining a final product which meets uniform quality and conforms to legal standards. Example for an ice cream mix is as follows:

Table 29

Sweet cream (25 % fat)	300 g
Fresh whole milk	500 g
Whole milk powder	80 g
Sugar	150 g
Stabiliser	2 g
Flavour	Few drops

Processing of Mix

Firstly all the liquid ingredients are heated. When the temperature reaches around 49 °C, the dry ingredients are added and mixed well. If gelatin is the stabiliser used, it is best added after thoroughly mixing with an equal quantity of sugar. Sodium alginate should not be added until temperature of the liquid material reaches at least 66 °C. (Colouring and flavouring agents are added at the time of freezing only). The ice cream mix thus obtained after mixing of the ingredients is then pasteurised either by batch or HTST methods.

Homogenisation

This is done to make a permanent and uniform suspension of fat by reducing the size of fat globules. Homogenisation is done at 60 - 65 °C.

Cooling and Ageing the Mix

The mix is cooled immediately after homogenisation to a temperature of 0 - 5 °C and is held at this temperature for 3-4 hours. Ageing improves the whipping capacity of mix and thus increases the over run of ice cream. If sodium alginate is used, no ageing is required.

Freezing the Mix

After ageing, colour and flavour are added and the mix is quickly frozen, being agitated to incorporate air and in such a way to produce and control the formation of small ice crystals. When the mix is frozen to semi solid consistency, it is drawn from the freezer at 4 to - 3 °C, in to packages and quickly transferred to hardening room. Ice cream can be frozen in batch freezers or continuous freezers.

Hardening and Storage

After drawn from the freezer with the packages, the ice cream is quickly transferred to the hardening room where the temperature is -18 °C or below. At the time of drawing from the freezer, ice cream is having a semi-fluid consistency. Freezing process continues in the hardening room without agitation and the ice cream is rendered stiff to hold its shape. After hardening ice cream may be immediately marketed or it may be stored for a week or two at the most. The storage temperature of ice cream is -18 to -23 °C.

Over Run in Ice Cream

It is the volume of ice cream obtained in excess of the volume of mix and is usually expressed as percentage. This increased volume is due to presence of air, which is incorporated during freezing.

$$\% \text{ over run is } = \frac{(\text{Volume of ice cream} - \text{Volume of mix})}{\text{Volume of mix}} \times 100$$

Normally the over run of ice cream ranges from 70 - 80 %.

Packaging of ice cream: Commonly used packaging material are paper or card board, plastic, fibre board coated with wax etc.

Chapter 18
CONCENTRATED AND DRIED MILK PRODUCTS

Condensed Milk

These are products obtained by evaporating a part of water from whole milk or skim milk with or without addition of sugar. The term condensed milk is commonly used for full cream sweetened condensed milk (Sweetened condensed whole milk). Evaporated milk is commonly used when referring to unsweetened condensed whole milk. Skimmed milk products are known as sweetened condensed skim milk and unsweetened condensed skim milk.

Table 30: Composition of Condensed Milk

	Condensed Milk	Evaporated Milk
Water (%)	26	31
Total solids (%)	74	69
Fat (%)	9	9
Milk SNF (%)	22	22
Protein (%)	8.3	8.3
Lactose (%)	12.2	12.2
Ash (%)	1.5	1.5
Sucrose (%)	43	—

Table 31

PFA Standards	Condensed Milk	Evaporated Milk
Milk fat (%) (Minimum)	9	8
Milk SNF (%) (Minimum)	31	26
Sugar (%) (Minimum)	40	—

Method of Preparation

Various steps in the preparation are:

Receiving Milk

Raw milk should be of high quality with regard to its heat stability. The heat stability of milk is determined by its acidity and mineral balance. Therefore a disturbed mineral balance causes objectionable heat coagulation. Alcohol test, which is an indication of high mineral content of milk should be negative for the milk which is used for condensed milk preparation.

Filtration

Milk is filtered to remove any visible foreign particles

Standardisation

It is done for adjusting fat and SNF ratio as 1:2.44

Pre Heating

A pre heating temperature of 80 - 85 °C is preferred to prevent age thickening (increase in viscosity during storage) and to destroy micro organisms and enzymes.

Addition of Sugar

Sugar is added at the end of condensing process. Liquid sugar (65 % sucrose) is pasteurised before addition.

Condensing

The basic principle of condensing consists removal of water from milk by boiling under partial vacuum at a low temperature till the desired concentration is achieved. Condensing is carried out in an evaporator. Use of vacuum evaporators prevents the heat damage of milk at high boiling temperatures. During condensing of milk the desired concentration of milk is checked by determining the density of a sample for which Baumay hydrometer is used.

Cooling and Crystallisation

Prompt cooling of the condensed milk is done to delay the chances of age thickening and discolouration and cooling is done to 30 °C. Crystallisation is the process of adding a small quantity of (0.1 - 0.3 %) very fine lactose crystals into the condensed milk for the formation of small crystals. This increases the smoothness of the product by avoiding formation of large ice crystals during storage (sandiness). After crystallisation, condensed milk is slowly cooled to a temperature of 15 °C.

Packaging

Commonly used packaging materials are barrels, drums, with polythene linings and tin containers for bulk packaging and tin cans for retail filling.

Storage

Condensed milk is preferably stored at 10 °C.

Uses

For reconstitution into sweet milk drinks, for preparation of tea/coffee, ice cream, confectionaries etc.

Khoa

It is a concentrated milk product obtained by heating milk in open vessels with continuous stirring so that water evaporates off leaving the solid portion. When the consistency becomes semi-solid it is sweetened by adding sugar. Composition of Khoa prepared form cow milk is Moisture 25.6 %, Fat 25.7 %, Protein 19.2 %, Lactose 25.5 % and Ash 3.8 %.

Method of Preparation

Milk taken in a open metallic vessel (Karahi) is boiled over a non smoky fire and is stirred continuously and vigorously in a circular motion by a stirrer. During this operation all parts of the pan with which the milk comes into contact are lightly scraped to prevent the milk from scorching. Constant evaporation of moisture take place and the milk thickens progressively. At certain concentration, there occurs an abrupt change in colour. Heating is continued thereafter with greater control and the speed of stirring cum scraping is increased. Soon the viscous mass reaches a semi solid consistency, shows signs of leaving the bottom and sides of the pan and starts sticking together. The fire is removed and the content is kneeded up and down into a single compact mass. Khoa is then cut into different sizes and shapes.

Packaging and Storage

Usually packaged in vegetable parchment paper, plastic film bags, laminated pouches, tin plate cans etc. Khoa has got low keeping quality at room temperature and refrigerated storage is recommended for better storage.

Khoa is used as base material for the preparation of sweets like Dooth peda, Gulabjamun, Peda, Burphi and for direct consumption.

Dried Milk Products

Drying is an important method of preserving food. Purpose of drying milk into milk powder are 1) To remove the moisture content of milk so as to reduce the bulkiness and there by saving in storage space and packaging cost. 2) To reduce the cost of transportation. 3) To improve the storage life of the product (due to low moisture content, bacterial growth is prevented). 4) To conserve the natural properties of the original raw material. 5) To conserve the seasonal surplus and for usage during lean seasons. Commonly used dried milk products include milk powder, baby food, malted milk food etc.

Milk Powder

Definition: Milk powder is a dried product prepared by evaporating water content of milk by heat or other suitable means to produce a solid product containing 5 % or less moisture. Whole milk or skim may be used for drying and the products thus obtained are called whole milk and skim milk powder respectively.

Table 32

PFA Standards	Whole Milk Powder	Skim Milk Powder
Moisture	5 % (minimum)	5 % (minimum)
Fat	26 % (minimum)	1.5 % (maximum)
Acidity (% of lactic acid)	1.2 (maximum)	1.5 (maximum)
SPC per gram	50,000 (maximum)	50,000 (maximum)
Solubility index		
for roller dried	15	15
for spray dried	2	2

Composition

Composition of whole milk powder and skim milk powder are as follows:

Table 33

Type of Powder	Moisture %	Fat %	Protein %	Lactose %	Ash %
WMP	2	27.5	26.4	38.2	5.9
SMP	3	.8	35.9	52.3	8

Method of Preparation

Basically there are two methods of drying such as heat drying and cold drying. Heat drying methods commonly used are roller drying and spray drying.

In roller drying milk is dried on large hollow cylinders heated to 150 °C by means of steam under pressure. Rotating rollers touches the pre heated milk so that a thin film of milk is formed on the rollers and is dried instantaneously. Dried film of milk is then scraped off from the roller by suitable blades before touching the milk again. Dried milk film is then ground to convert into powder and the dry powder thus obtained is sieved and suitably packed.

Advantages of Roller Drying

1. Relatively low capital and operational cost
2. Plant is movable and occupies less space
3. Easy to handle
4. Suitable for small quantities of milk

Disadvantages

1. Powder is less soluble
2. Produce a cooked flavour to reconstituted milk

In spray drying milk is sprayed as minute droplets into a large chamber, with a current of hot air (130 - 140 °C). The water content is removed very fast and fine powder settles at the bottom of the chamber and is then continuously removed before charring out of over heating.

Advantages

1. Spray dried powder is superior in quality with respect to colour, flavour and solubility in water.
2. Economical for large scale operation

Disadvantage
1. Involve large capital investment
2. Sophisticated instrumentation

Packaging

Commonly done in fibre board cartons, polythene bags, tin cans, plastic bottles etc.

Storage

High storage temperatures decreases the keeping quality of milk powder. Therefore temperatures lower than 24 °C is preferred. Refrigeration should be used for long storage in warm climate. To ensure maximum keeping quality, milk powder should be stored in vapour proof, moisture proof and sealed packages in cool and dry places.

Uses

Milk powder is widely used for reconstituting milk, as a whitener for tea and coffee, as a constituent of various baby foods and for preparation of various milk products.

Other Dried Milk Products

Infant Milk Food

It is the product obtained by drying milk with the addition of specific carbohydrates like cane sugar, dextrose and dextrin, maltose and Iron salts, vitamins etc. Example of infant milk food is Lactogen, Cerelac etc.

Table 34

PFA Standard	
Moisture (maximum)	5 %
Milk fat	18 - 28 %
Milk protein (Min.)	20 %
Total carbohydrates (Min.)	35 %
Total ash (Max.)	8.5 %
Iron (Min.)	4 mg/100 g
Vitamin A (Min)	15 IU/g
SPC per gram (Max.)	50,000
Solubility index	
Roller dried	15
Spray dried	2

Malted Milk Food

It is the product obtained by mixing milk powder with malt extract and cereal grain flour or drying milk with these ingredients so as to secure complete hydrolysis of starchy material.

Table 35

PFA Standard	
Moisture (Max.)	5 %
Milk fat (Min.)	7 % (Dry matter basis)
Total ash (Max.)	5 % (- do -)
Acid insoluble ash (Max.)	0.1 % (- do -)
Nitrogen (Min.)	2 % (- do -)
SPC per gram (Max.)	50,000
Coliform count / gram (Max.)	10
Solubility (Min.)	80 %

Chapter 19

MISCELLANEOUS DAIRY PRODUCTS AND BY-PRODUCTS

Indigenous Milk Sweets

Indigenous milk based sweets or traditional milk sweets are those originated in India. A significant proportion of milk has been used in India for preparing a wide variety of dairy sweets. In the process, the basic limitation of milk - its perishable nature - has been tastefully overcomed, because its processing also aims to extend the shelf life of milk. Some of the common and popular milk sweets are Peda, Gulab Jamun, Burfi, Rossogolla, etc. Method of preparation of some of these milk sweets are given below.

Peda

It is khoa based milk sweet. Ingredients used are:

1. *Khoa*: 225 g
2. *Sugar*: 75 g
3. *Pista (optional)*: A few pieces
4. *Cardamom (optional)*: A few sticks
5. *Silver paper (optional)*: One leaf

Break freshly made khoa into bits. Mix sugar into it. Put into open vessel and cook over a very slow non-smoky fire, stirring continuously with a ladle. Add crushed cardamom if desired. When mixture is ready (mixture form balls when tested), pour into a tray and leave to cool and set. Peda is now ready. Decorate if desired with silver paper and sliced pista. Cut into required size and shape to serve.

Gulab Jamun

This is also a khoa based milk sweet. Ingredients required are:

1. *Khoa*: 300 g
2. *Maida*: 35 g
3. *Baking powder*: 1 or 2 tsp
4. *Sugar*: 1 Kg
5. *Water*: 1 Kg
6. *Ghee*: 500 g

Break freshly made khoa into bits. Mix baking powder into the maida separately. Add this mixture to the broken khoa and mix again. Now start kneeding by adding small quantities of water until uniform dough is obtained. Consistency of the dough should be such that when made into small balls it has a smooth uncracked surface. Mean while dissolve all the sugar in water and boiled the solution till a 2- string - consistency is obtained. Now make the balls and fry in sufficient ghee in a shallow pan so as to immerse the ball completely during frying. The ball should be neither over nor under fried. They should be deep brown in colour. Remove the balls and put them into syrup immediately, pressing them down into sugar syrup for some time so that it soaks in. Keep Gulab Jamun at room temperature for at least 10 -12 hours before serving.

Burfi

This is another khoa based sweet. There are three types of burfi such as plain burfi, chocolate burfi and coconut burfi.

Ingredients

1. *Khoa*: 250 g
2. *Sugar*: 75 g

Break khoa into bits and add sugar in to it. Put in open over gentle heat and stir vigorously with a ladle. Collect the mixture into a tray when all the sugar has dissolved. This is plain burfi. If chocolate is added into above mixture the product is called chocolate burfi. If coconut (grated fine and dried) is mixed with plain burfi, it is called coconut burfi. Suitable colour can be added if desired.

Kalakand

Ingredients

1. *Milk*: 1 Kg
2. *Sugar*: 60 g
3. *Citric acid*: 1 or 2 g
4. *Pista (optional)* : A few pieces
5. *Silver paper (optional)* : 1 leaf
6. *Cardamom*: a few sticks.

Boil milk in a open vessel placed over a non-smoky fire. Stir continuously with a ladle. After 10 -15 minutes add to it, the required amount of citric acid. This will partially coagulate the milk. At this time vigorous stirring is required to obtain a product of good quality. When a semi solid stage is reached add sugar and stir well. Also add fresh cardamom if desired. Remove from fire after 5 minutes. This product is set in a greasy tray and allowed to cool. Kalakand is now ready. Decorate if desired with silver paper and Pista. Cut in to required size and shape to serve.

Sandesh

This is a chhana based milk sweet.

Ingredients

1. *Chhana*: 250 g
2. *Sugar*: 75 g
3. *Flavour (optional)* : a few drops
4. *Cardamom (optional)* : a few sticks.

Break freshly made chhana into bits. Mix sugar into it. Put the mixture in a open vessel and heat on a slow fire with continuous stirring. Add crushed cardamom if desired. When the mixture is ready to torm balls, pour into a tray and allowed to cool. Sandesh is now ready. It is cut into desired size and shape.

Rossogolla

This is also a chhana based milk sweet.

Ingredients

1. *Chhana*: 200 g
2. *Maida (optional)* : 8g
3. *Sugar*: 250 g
4. *Water*: 1 Kg.
5. *Flavour*: a few drops.

Break the above quantity of chhana into bits and start kneeding. If required a small quantity of maida may be added to avoid cracks in the finished Rossogolla. The consistency of the kneeded mass should be such that when made into small balls, it has a smooth surface with no signs of cracks. Meanwhile dissolve all the sugar in water and boil the solution. Now make the balls of chhana and put them gently in the boiling sugar syrup for the cooking process. The heating should be so controlled that the balls are constantly covered with foam. After 5-10 minutes the balls will swell and colour of balls will darken slightly. The finished Rossogolla should normally be ready after 20 -2 5 minutes. After cooling, sprinkle flavour to serve.

Chhana-Kheer

It is a chhana based milk sweet. Ingredients for preparation include:

1. *Milk*: 1 Kg
2. *Chhana*: 150 g
3. *Sugar*: 40 g
4. *Flavour (optional)* : Few drops
5. *Dry nuts*: Few pieces.

Cut the chhana into small cubes. Boil the milk and reduce into half of its original volume. Add sugar and boil further till its original volume is reduced to 1/3. Then add the pieces of chhana and continue heating gently until sugar has penetrated into chhana cubes. When cooled, sprinkle flavour on the chhana cubes. If desired decorate with dry nuts.

Chhana-Murki

This is also a chhana based sweet. Required ingredients are:

1. *Chhana:* 250 g
2. *Sugar:* 125 g
3. *Water:* 45 g
4. *Flavour:* Few drops
5. *Dry nuts:* Few pieces.

Dissolve sugar in water and boil the mixture until it has a three string consistency. Cut the chhana into small cubes and put them into the prepared sugar syrup in an open vessel. Boil the mixture for 5 minutes and remove the fire. Allow the contents to cool. Stir the cubes till the entire sugar is uniformly coated around them. Sprinkle flavour and decorate with dry nuts.

Pantooa

This is Khoa cum chhana based sweet. Ingredients are:

1. *Khoa:* 300g
2. *Chhana:* 300 g
3. *Baking powder:* 1 or 2 tsp.
4. *Maida:* 35 g
5. *Sugar:* 1 Kg
6. *Water:* 1 Kg
7. *Ghee:* 500 g

Break all the Khoa and chhana into small bits. Mix baking powder with maida separately. Add this mixture to the broken Khoa and Chhana. Start kneeding adding small quantities of water until a uniform dough is obtained. There after the preparatory steps are similar to that of Gulab Jamun.

Dairy By-products

A dairy by-product may be defined as a product of commercial value produced during the manufacture of a main product. *E.g.,* Skim milk, Buttermilk, Whey, Casein etc. Skim milk is the byproduct obtained during the separation of milk into cream. Skim milk can be used for preparing casein, fermented milk, skim milk powder etc.

Buttermilk is obtained after churning cream into butter and can be used for purposes like preparation of fermented milk, soft cheese etc. Whey is the liquid portion drained out of coagulated milk during preparation of cheese or paneer. This can be used for preparing various whey beverages, whey paste, lactose etc.

Casein

Casein is the milk protein otherwise known as coagulated protein of milk, which contribute about 80 % of milk protein. Casein is commercially prepared from skim milk. According to the mode of usage, casein can be broadly classified into industrial casein and edible casein. Industrial casein refers to the casein, which is mainly used in the industry for making plastic, adhesives, paint etc. It can be either acid casein or rennet casein. The casein precipitated by various acids is called acid casein and that precipitated by rennet is called rennet casein.

Edible Casein

Defined as casein which has been isolated from skim milk by taking special precautions to ensure its suitability for use in food and pharmaceutical preparations. This precautions are concerned with strict control of:

1. Quality of raw material.
2. Use of standard techniques of production.
3. Maintenance of strict hygienic conditions of production.
4. Packaging and storage under approved conditions.

Edible casein is used in various food products like ice cream, coffee whitener, imitation milk, whipping powders etc.

Method of Preparation

Various steps in the preparation of casein include :

1. Receiving skim milk
2. Precipitating
3. Draining and washing
4. Pressing
5. Milling and spreading
6. Drying

7. Grinding

8. Packaging.

Whey

The whey obtained as a by product of cheese or paneer industry is used in the production of fermented beverages both alcoholic and non-alcoholic, condensed whey, whey protein concentrates, whey paste etc. Whey beverages are obtained by fermenting whey with suitable cultures of yeast or bacteria. Yeast produces alcoholic whey beverage Example is Whevit. Non-alcoholic or acidic whey beverages are obtained by fermenting whey with suitable lactic acid bacteria, which convert lactose into lactic acid producing acid taste.

Condensed whey is made evaporating the liquid portion of the whey using vacuum evaporators. If sugar is added it is called sweetened condensed whey and otherwise plain condensed whey. Whey protein concentrates includes soluble and coagulated whey protein. The technique of electro-dialysis, gel filtration and reverse osmosis are recently used for the preparation of whey protein concentrates. Whey paste is prepared by pre concentrating a mixture of whey and skim milk in vacuum evaporator and adding sugar, butter and cream so as to obtain 65 % total solids in the finished product. Lactose is another by product commercially prepared from cheese whey through evaporation and crystallisation and is used for preparing humanised milk, infant foods and pharmaceutical preparations.

INDEX